TODDLER
DISCIPLINE:

The Effective Strategies to Tame
Tantrums. A Guide to help Children
developing Self-Discipline through a
positive parenting approach.

MARLA CALLORY & SUSY MASON

Table of Contents

Introduction

Discipline is essential for all toddler, and we can consider it as the basis of education, though we wonder who is the most responsible for teaching and practicing it. Parents often say that teachers are the ones who should impose the basis of the discipline and to carry them out in the classroom. On the contrary, teachers affirm that this must be done at home, and many times this leads to the child being expected to show a behavior that has not been taught either at home or in the school.

Disciplining a toddler is never easy. It is rather challenging because, to effectively discipline your toddler, you must have a thorough understanding of their state of mental development. A child between the ages of one and three doesn't have the ability to think rationally the way an older child does. This mental maturity doesn't allow them to understand or remember the rules you set. Even if they understand the rules, they might not be able to retain them for long. Apart from this, their ability to empathize with others, along with their instinct of self-preservation, is still in the stages of construction. Their understanding of logic, along with the consequences of their actions, is still in the primitive stages.

You must understand that your toddler is still in the initial phases of developing their sense of self and will want to do everything for themself. They might want to do things that they aren't fully capable of doing yet. This, in turn, might be a source of frustration. This, when combined with the fact that they aren't fully able to communicate verbally, means that they will start venting out their frustrations by throwing tantrums and by indulging in unruly behavior.

Another thing you must keep in mind while dealing with a toddler is that it might not be their intention to misbehave. In fact, the way they behave is essentially their response to a situation. They are responding in the best way their underdeveloped maturity allows them to. So, you must be quite empathetic and understanding whenever you're dealing with your toddler. You must be aware of all that your toddler is going through along with their developmental growth. By becoming aware of these factors, it becomes easier to respond to them while disciplining them.

It's important that we introduce an understanding of positive discipline before approaching behavior. This book will teach you what positive discipline is, from when to apply it to how to do it properly.

Positive discipline is a new method that is used to look after babies and children in a different way by using a different point of view. While in the traditional discipline we speak of punishing wrong behavior, in the positive discipline, we keep in mind the type of adult we want to create and what would be the reaction of society to that mistake.

Consistency is the key to successful discipline. If you say you're going to do something if your child acts up, then you must follow through the minute it happens. Often if a child acts up and you wait half a day to get back to punishment, they may have forgotten what they did, or they may not connect the punishment and discipline with their misbehavior. Keep it consistent and administer the discipline and punishment the moment the misbehavior occurs. Remember to set boundaries, stay consistent, and practice all discipline with your love and patience. Once a toddler learns they will be disciplined for bad behavior, they will change their ways.

A better approach to disciplining your child is to use techniques that foster their ability to make moral judgments about right and wrong for themself. My main objective in here is that all readers become aware that discipline is not only to punish toddler and get them to do what we want, but many other aspects are covered as capacities or skills are created respecting their characteristics individual; In addition, values such as respect, tolerance, responsibility are fostered, it is for all the above that discipline is not only crucial in childhood but will also help in adult life.

There are essential aspects that should be considered when applying the discipline, in addition to some strategies and steps that guide us to establish discipline with appropriate norms and limits, which you'll know as you enter the reading.

Remember that discipline isn't only punishment but as mentioned before, it's a process that involves many aspects.

Parents must remain calm, sound, and be in control emotionally. Anyone who has a kid in their life will have undoubtedly had that moment when they feel they have lost all control when that kid throws a killer tantrum when you wonder whatever happened to the right parenting skills that you thought you had just a few minutes before. The good news is it's normal if your toddler throws tantrums. Likewise, if you feel as if you're struggling as a parent to deal with these tantrums, that's normal too. None of us are automatically born with good parenting skills, and it's only through advice, guidance, and trial and error that we will ever have the parenting skills we need to survive for the discipline of children.

Chapter 1: Understanding Life from a Toddler's Point of View

Do you remember the imaginary friend you used to keep in your closet when you were a child? Do you remember the innocent outlook on the world? Do you remember how much fun it was playing in the mud? No?   Well,

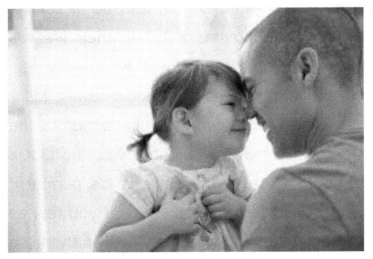

maybe it's time you remember.

A toddler hardly ever does something knowing that it's wrongs the first time. They have been in this world for far fewer years than we have and it's our job to teach them these things.

Learning by Example

Things need to be explained and made clear to toddlers. Looking at the world from their point of view will make this so much easier. Toddlers get engrossed in the present and don't think about the consequences. They live in the past and the present but rarely take the time to look at the future and what consequences their actions will bring them.

Here are a few tips to help see things from a toddler's point of view and why each tip is useful:

Consider what works from their point of view

Toddlers whine, cry, and yell for attention. Why? Because it works for them. To them, it's what gets you to give them attention. They don't care whether it's good or bad. It gets you to stop what you're doing and take a minute to listen to them or pick them up. They are smarter than what we give them credit for. This is something that I will repeat multiple times because it's something we shouldn't forget.

Acknowledge what they are feeling

Talking about feelings can be tough as an adult but young children don't really care. They don't yet understand why they should share their feelings and why not, so they are in an oversharing stage of their life that doesn't seem to end for a very long time. At least, that's what it feels like.

It's good to talk about feelings with them and to acknowledge what they are feeling. "I understand that you're angry," or "I know that you don't want to stop playing with your dolls" are good examples. When anything or anyone goes against a tot's wishes it's as if the entire world is turned against them and that is when they start acting up.

Letting them know that you understand all this makes things a little easier for them. Try to relate to them as well. Try using words like "I don't want playtime to end either."

Limited speech

Try to turn the time back in your mind and remember the vocabulary you possessed at the age of your toddler. It's not very big, is it? Try thinking of it as an Italian trying to speak to a German. Both parties will get flustered when they don't understand each other. A toddler wants you to read their mind and know exactly where their vocabulary ends and where you should start using your own initiative.

Try finding the hints your child drops when they don't understand you. They may tilt their head to one side or might furrow their brow. Try explaining something in a simpler way to them.

"I see this one way and no way else"

Toddlers have a way of keeping one view and one view only. Say they want a cookie and you're telling them that they can't get it because it's bad for them. In their minds, they are convinced that they need the cookie and don't understand that it's bad for them. They are still learning that there are different sides to a story and not just theirs. Be patient and try to explain it to them to the best of your abilities.

Set an example

It is vital to lead by example. Toddlers take on a lot of traits, good and bad, from their parents. At this tender age, they are like a sponge and take in anything and everything they possibly can. Yelling and raging will teach your child that it's alright to do this. No one wants a screaming tot and I can promise you that is exactly what will happen if you give them the tiniest inkling that it's okay to behave in such a manner.

Setting an example might not put you in their shoes, but it will give them some shoes to step into. Kids are easily manipulatable and can be influenced quite easily. They will adapt to their surroundings because it's part of their instincts and they don't understand the world in the same way adults do. They will take on the personality of whatever they need to survive.

There is nothing a child idolizes more than their parents and what better examples to follow? There will be times when you feel like you want to strangle the kid but remember that you're an adult and you need to set the example. Also, if the child sees you acting that way when there is trouble, it will give them the idea that it's okay to act like that around other children as well.

Freeze, Fight, or Flight

When you're putting yourself in their shoes and thinking like they are thinking, how do you react to a raging parent? Freeze, fight, or flight? None of these are remotely the reaction you are looking for in a child. Either they freeze and they shut you out entirely, fight and make you even angrier because, let's face it, if you do it, they will want to do it too, or choose flight. No parent wants a child to run away from them and hide. It goes against every paternal instinct we have.

Tots will mirror our actions and if we are handling it calmly, so will they. Most kids will stop what they are doing and listen. But remember, just because you're being calm about the situation does not mean you can't be strict or firm. Sometimes the tot will need a firm voice to slow them down or coax them out of their shell so they will listen.

Good leadership skills are often established as a result of these events, and the only way to strengthen your effective child management skills is to regularly cope with such tantrums and get the opportunity to know what works better for your toddler." It will also help with all the training skills in parenting strategies for children. Often, it's easy to lose out on hints and signs on what could set your child off. Keeping a diary of what leads to these baby tantrums is a fantastic way to help you identify any potential areas of trouble. But don't try to avoid those situations. That just prolongs the inevitable. Instead, keep your expectations consistent, and your child will eventually realize that there is no point in tantrums about this.

Along with patience, putting yourself in their place is the other parenting tip for kids' discipline skills that you'll need to ensure you get the best out of your child. Obviously, that is very difficult to achieve because we are adults; we all know what is risky, and we understand that when we want them, we cannot have those things that we want. But a kid cannot understand any of those things, and you can't just use logic or talk to them about the reason. But please don't bother. You have the final say about what your child is doing or not getting, and they must understand that.

Realize instead that this is just a phase. Even as a kid, you should be setting a few basic rules in their very early stages of life. Not too many, a good figure is around 4 or 5. When setting these rules, one thing you should remember is that you need to be firm with them. If you set rules, then you're supposed to stand by them; otherwise, there isn't much use. Explain to your kid what the rules are, and then, whenever they break one go over the rule again.

Also, your kid should realize you're the parent; they need to do what you're saying. Kids are well behaved as well as badly behaved at times. When they are well behaved, then give praise to your child, and this will reinforce that they will be praised with good behavior but disciplined with bad behavior. If your kid misbehaves, then act with a voice of firm authority. For example, if they are asked to turn off the TV and they won't, be firm when you say, "do as I say," don't be angry about it. If the discipline of your kid doesn't work and your kid is defiant, don't give in. If you send them this, it's a sure sign the next time they're only going to be more stubborn and get their way. Time-out is one effective form of discipline for the toddler. If your kid is defiant, then you can send them to a place or a time-out room. Let your kid know they're going to have to sit still in time-out so they can think about their behavior. Explain to your kid that they will remain in their room until they are ready to come and talk about their behavior with you. This is a simple but prevalent form of discipline, and it's effective.

It's no surprise that problems for infants are mostly behavioral. Toddlers are at the point where they learn a language, develop interpersonal skills, and assert their independence in their lives. Tact and kindness are, of course, two things that do not exist in their vocabulary yet. So, how does a parent treat common problems with the infants? By learning the methods of manipulation and adapt to it. Aside from expert strategies, you can develop your own strategy to fix problems with children. Here are some simple, workable tips you could try.

Place Rules -Teach the concept of good and bad behavior to your toddler. You do this by recognizing the good they are doing and correcting the bad.

Be consistent - Once you have come up with a rule, never bend it. If you do, you teach your child to be a potential lawbreaker, an offender, or an exception to every rule.

Give instructions which are clear and straightforward - Remember your kid has a very limited vocabulary, so choose simple but firm commands when giving instructions. **"Stop"** and **"Don't"** are two verbs which should be of very good service to you.

Persevere in tackling the problems of your baby in all ways. With positive reinforcement and constant reminders, your kid won't be a terrible two-year-old. If you're a parent of infants, you know how daily life can be exhausting. One minute your little one can be as cute as a bug and then just a few moments later rapidly morph into a holy terror. There are some basic parenting strategies you can use to help make life more manageable when you have kids. Knowing how to parent your children wisely is important, so that that you and your children are happier and healthier. Rather than being overwhelmed by the responsibilities and challenges that parents are constantly presented with, they need to understand that "wisely choosing your parenting battles" is very good advice and be rest assured of your expectations and requirements and learn to enjoy this special time with your children.

Tantrums are tough. There is no doubt about it. It's tough for you as a parent to watch your child experience a meltdown. It's tough for your child to be the one melting down in the first place. When you're dealing with a child throwing a tantrum, you may be quick to feel like you should just give in, hoping to avoid the problem altogether, but that isn't going to help here. Rather, when you're dealing with your child throwing a tantrum, you should remind yourself of the one fact that was repeated throughout this book. Make it your new mantra. Print it out and put it on sticky notes everywhere throughout your home to remind you of the truth:

Your child isn't giving you a hard time. They are having a hard time.

Let this be your life's motto and you'll be able to keep your cool, even when you find your child melting down in the middle of the grocery store for the third time that day. Children are rough to parents but growing up is tough too. Remember, growing up is all about learning to see a world that you are entirely unfamiliar with. Everyone goes through it—none of us are born knowing how the world works, and that is okay.

Allow yourself to find the mindset of recognizing that you can, discipline your child without punishment, and that discipline is what you should aim for.

A small child, by definition, is someone who gets up and walks. The word 'boy' is a combination of the Scottish words toddler and waddle and refers to the awkward way babies get up and walk around like drunken sailors, with their legs spread apart, their arms raised in the air and lots of jerking.

As you'll soon discover, there are many wonderful aspects of life with a young child, including their boundless energy, their passion for exploring the world, their spontaneous expressions of affection, and their witty mischief and leaving childhood behind as they continue to become an independent child.

As your sense of self and limits begin to take shape, there will be times when your child is likely to throw tantrums, refuse to eat what was set before them, stiffen, and firmly resist being tied to their stroller or car seat, to be extremely upset that you can't read their mind and refuse to share their toys with their playmates. These are all typical behaviors for this incredible and unique stage in human life.

When it comes to discipline, parents face an avalanche of disparate expert advice that can be puzzling, contradictory, and sometimes simply impossible to follow. Can parents bribe, reward, spank, neglect, offer consequences, or order a timeout? Does gentle discipline mean allowing children to rule the chicken coop? If parents use threats, distractions, games, graphics, timers, count to three or "the perfect look"

No wonder so many of the parents are confused, frustrated, and paralyzed. No wonder parents are losing confidence.

Young children, in particular, are likely to push limits. It is their job as active learners and explorers, and it is appropriate for them to develop. It's a defining attribute of their intense mix of emotions as they seek to be more autonomous. Successful mentoring gives children the security and comfort they need in order to thrive. When it comes to working limitations, kids don't have to test them as often. They trust their parents and caregivers, and therefore their world. They feel more free and calmer and can focus on significant things: playing, learning, socializing, and being happy children.

The parent's emotional state almost always determines the child's reaction when setting limits. If we lack consistency and confidence, lose our patience, or are nervous, stressed, exhausted, or irritated, this will annoy our children and possibly lead to more unwanted behavior. In our children's eyes, we are gods, and our feelings always set the tone. With that understanding, it's easy to see why discipline struggles can become a vicious, discouraging circle.

All too often, however, we continue to treat our babies and toddlers as empty, unconscious, and incapable of understanding us or communicating with us. Instead, we could expect our children to be able to handle adult situations (such as an afternoon shopping trip at the mall) with a mental maturity and emotional self-control that they have not yet developed. These imprecise perceptions can lead parents in an unproductive direction, especially with regard to discipline issues.

Ultimately, the big step to successful discipline is to get rid of the short-term fix tricks, cheats, and all other tactics of manipulation and just be honest with our babies and infants (what a concept!).

It can also be argued that the influence of society is powerful. Parents will judge themselves by how others are dealing with parenthood. At the same time, it's easier even for young children to be exposed to violence and negative influences which will later affect their outlook on life.

As a parent, this can be particularly frustrating. Guiding your child is difficult enough without outside influences adjusting their responses, particularly those that are beyond your control.

The result is often visible in the number of children which are experiencing social issues. Some children are unruly, difficult to control, and even aggressive despite the best intentions of parents. Many will say the child simply needs discipline, but there is generally more to parenting than disciplining your child. This is, perhaps, the most difficult challenge.

Discipline is essential to ensure your child knows what is right and wrong, and it can also teach what is socially acceptable behavior. Unfortunately, this standard is often different depending upon where the family lives. Discipline must be balanced against guidance, love, and nurturing; these are the things which will help your child grow into a healthy and well-adjusted young person.

Parents themselves will often feel the pressure to "get it right." It is common, especially for new parents, to feel that they are being judged by other parents. School and even playgroups are one place where a parent would hope to gain support and be able to assess the milestones their child should be able to reach. Yet, frequently, this is one of the places where a parent is judged the most.

Advances in medical science also play their part. It's often possible to diagnose a child with Autism or Attention Deficit Hyperactivity Disorder (ADHD), and whilst this should increase understanding from others it, often invokes a negative reaction. There are two reasons for this: others will either feel your child simply has a label to justify their behavior, or they won't fully understand the condition and simply keep their children away from yours. Both scenarios can make it harder to get the parenting balance right.

Finally, it's useful to consider time and family ties. Modern society often requires both parents to work in order to survive, leaving your child in the hands of someone else whose parenting style may not be the same as yours. This can make it difficult to enforce your expectations. This is complicated further when families separate and stepfamilies are created. Although all children should be treated equally, this isn't always the case.

The result of all these pressures and the limited time you have available for your child often means it's easier to discipline than to guide. A child's natural enthusiasm and energy can simply be too much at the end of a long day, and while snapping at your child may seem like the easiest option, it simply makes being a good parent harder.

Chapter 2: Discipline for toddlers

To become a socially acceptable person, an infant must be taught how to control itself, especially the less acceptable aspects of its personality. A child cannot simply be left to do as they pleases, and it is the responsibility of the parents to assert control over their children in the form of discipline, to demonstrate that they approve of certain types of behavior and disapprove of others. Whether and why this power is applied depends to some degree on the child's perceptions of the parents, and the way they controlled themselves. It also depends on the expectations of the whole of their

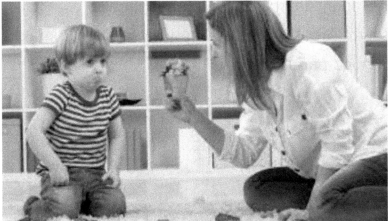

socie ty and on the particular culture the child is born into. For example, some communities exercise a firmer discipline than the traditional American one, and this can lead to conflict in the minds of certain children in ethnic minority groups. Parents should try to understand why the infant has bad behaviors. It might not be just bad temper or naughtiness, but it might be this:

They are tired and want some relaxing.

They are not well or perhaps are sickening of some illness.

They are jealous of the newborn babies, or in any way feel left out.

They are worried about some new experience, like starting school or going to the hospital.

They're lonely, and they want something to be busy with and involved in.

Older brothers or sisters tease them, or playmates.

They feel insecure and test their parents' affection.

Remedies to Treat Challenges in Toddlers

Letting them mingle with other kids.

Finding others for them to play with.

Attending Mother and Toddler Groups.

Organizing birthday parties and other children's trips.

Letting them go to a playgroup.

Kids Dance Lessons.

Public library sessions and other social activities.

All these activities help in curbing bad behavior in children as they are non-confrontational and emotional.

Making Them Aware of the Need for Others to Consider This involves teaching and applying good social behaviors, such as table manners, politeness, and good personal hygiene, so as not to offend others. A snack bar or restaurant visit maybe a treat, but it will also provide valuable social training. Encourage the kid to share their possessions and take turns with their mother, teachers, and other adults in mind. It's also important to be careful with your behavior and make sure your kid isn't slipping into a biting habit. Never bite your child back; this only teaches them that adults can bite even though children don't have to. It's also good to avoid playing biting games with him, including trying to bite their toes etc., while discovering that biting isn't the right behavior. Toddlers like to see balanced displays of frustration from their parents and then see a skillful resolution of disputes. This is the way they learn to do it on their own. Its aim is to play fair before them. They keep an eye on your reactions.

Using a variety of forms of punishment

So, avoiding negative behavior in children is about using a variety of forms of punishment before you find one that fits best for your child. Here are five methods of discipline that you can try with your child, hopefully bringing a swift end to their bad behavior:

Preventing Issues Before

Seeking a constructive approach to punishment is a smart way to avoid the development of negative habits and conflicts first. Take away temptations that are too big for your kid, such as putting markers or your makeup case out of your kid's reach if you don't want them to use these items, or to not keep chips or sweets in the house if your request for them not to eat these items before dinner is ignored. Set your child up for success and avoid a lot of bad behavior and drama.

Give Children Options

Give your kid the chance to pick from two different options to give them more control over the situation where possible. For example, if your kid refuses to get clad in the morning, giving them two clothes to choose from can take away the struggle of getting dressed and remove the negative behavior. By giving them choices, letting your child feel like they have some control, makes cooperation natural and simple.

I DON'T UNDERSTAND

If your child ever speaks to you inappropriately, simply proclaim incomprehension. Look at them with a puzzled face - as though they were using a foreign language - and plainly say: 'I can't understand you while you're talking like that.' Though your child is crying, do the same thing except then say: "I don't understand 'Whinese.' Can you talk in English, please?" And ignore your child before they respond to you in a more acceptable fashion. They will soon learn that speaking to you in a "natural" tone of reverence is the best way to get your attention and eventually get an answer from you. Do you want to try more disciplinary techniques with your child?

Chapter 3: Montessori Disciplines

Maria Montessori felt the youngster's ability of consideration will build up throughout their dealing using substances inside activities as it can help in their capacity to focus and consequently establishing their persona. With improved immersion, the youngster will be soon wealthier and much more regulated, which almost certainly describes a kid might be 'normalized' when they're earnestly engaged with purposeful pursuits. This is also a result of how a kid should visit a point when they are soon quite curious about something and also might require to governs it. It's most likely what Montessori phrases that while the youngster's painful and sensitive phases come then they will have motivation to know something. The truth is that Montessori considered that "if kiddies don't disclose an urge to operate incrementally, the error is located not only from the kiddies, though, in exactly the mode of introducing exactly the issues to be researched. Hence, she ardently believed it is of extreme significance that the educator knows that the various requirements of their students so as to divert the interest of their youngster. Also, to concentrate on what demands as "if kids are exhausted, inattentive and uncomprehending it's as the processes for instruction utilized current insuperable hurdles to this 'spontaneous' operation of their youngster's intellect.

For your little one to know how to be self-discipline, still, another element that's only as essential since the right collection of substances to your youngster is the fact that the youngster needs to be directed to achieve liberty. Montessori considered the youngster must receive the chance to operate well with substances from the surroundings. It's essential as kids learn through the usage of these senses; they will need to govern matters. It's futile to allow a kid a high-value toy that goes onto a unique and won't permit the kid to socialize with this anyhow foresee it. The youngster isn't going to learn whatever. For this reason, parents must pick out their toys to the kiddies precisely, together with all the targets of mastering expertise at heart.

Still another variable is that the youngster has to build up the will. The youngster could be permitted to select which task they want to do. As they're motivated for the task, they will possess the attention to focus on it, ergo finish the endeavor. It may aid in the creation of their self-discipline since Montessori considered that every child includes an all organic inner impulse that'll guide them purposeful pursuits like replicating the actions as a way to correct the art learned. This replicated action can aid the kid to add control within them and also the environmental surroundings. They're learning how to make their conclusions about things such as what they want. It enables them to accept responsibility due to their actions merely. The game which they undertake may allow them to know that the constraints of actuality, thus causing them into self-knowledge, self-possession along with self-discipline. Self-discipline is just a rather crucial feature for your kid to accomplish, so to allow them personally to produce elements like the strength of concentration and attention and also the liberty to execute imagination and work while to ease finding out.

For your little one to acquire self-discipline, they should supply work. It's thus the educator's or so the caregiver's occupation to choose the clues about the little one regarding what experts suggest and exactly what activities may appeal to them at a time. At high temperature which suits them personally, they'll have the ability to select the experience that interests them, thus allowing them to revolve around the job available. The youngster must not engage in numerous activities as to confound their intellect and interrupt his or her development. Ergo, it's necessary for your educator along with your physician to know the youngster and be in a position to reply professionally. While the youngster enjoys governing matters and learns very best through drama, the task posed needs to be enjoyment and also attractive to the kid. Just this manner, would the little one be in a position to come up with their self-discipline because they knowingly call themself into their preferred section of the job.

Freedom at the Montessori classroom can be misunderstood not solely by your parents, but additionally by a few educators. That which we will need to bear in mind is the fact that in the Montessori position of perspective, freedom isn't the thing to get when you want it without consideration of others. Additionally, it doesn't follow the sole manner that the youngster might be resourceful is always to be authorized to accomplish anything they select without the constant parameters along with guidance in your adult while in the space. For independence to get the job done efficiently and invisibly, it's to serve inside the business tips of the subject. Discipline doesn't indicate having to bow to the will of someone. Independence and discipline are just two sides of the same coin.

Freedom is your capacity to avoid, believe, and earn an option with the exclusion of some specified actions. Will-power is making correct decisions while valuing the ecosystem, and also the rights of others. Yes, outline all this to them to allow them to grow healthy, which makes the youngster behave and receive chances to blossom. But this doesn't mean the educator abdicates accountability. Although, on the contrary, it places better responsibility for the educator.

Even the teacher gets the obligation of establishing business parameters, and parameters over the flexibility could use appropriately. This is a difficult job, especially if the educator cannot accurately interpret the Montessori independence and subject heritage within their mind. Also, all the educators have to do is put out clear expectations and guidelines to where flexibility could occur. Kids are likewise proficient manipulators, and up until now in their lives they thought there were no expectations of them. So, they will try to observe how they can drive and transform the guidelines to suit themselves. It's for that particular reason why the rules and expectations must get made evident firmly at the start of the school season.

Each of these includes the educator to become vigilant and consistent. They don't need to be tagged "hard" or "mean." first, let them figure out how to stay consistent while finding joy as well. Some educators find that particularly hard. While attempting to dictate, a few educators neglect to show concern or care. Some are too hard on kids, thinking if this isn't maintained the child will believe there is "wiggle room" to violate the principles. If they believe this then they are fighting their freedom and also subjecting them to coercion in a year long-term.

So, how can we maintain freedom while ensuring a healthy environment for growth? How can we walk the fine line to equilibrium and keep the suitable freedom and subject?

Below are a few pointers that have work effectively

Foster liberty in the area usual manners.

Permit freedom to proceed, to convey, to opt for exercise, to do the job along with others.

Supply constraints that offer lessons on leadership in this sensation of freedom.

Encouraging actions that don't harm others or interfere with other's matters.

If the decision they make suits their personality and helps them move forward, then it should be supported.

The decision, the youngster, might utilize cloth with the objective of which it was meant, right in regard.

During more engaging activities certain things need to be restricted, perhaps a certain way of acting or a range of materials or maybe a toy so that the child can perform at their best.

Not one of those is news to the more knowledgeable Montessori instructors. Though, frequent reminders are useful for the encouragement of many educators, notably those who always battle with the idea of independence and subject. Same as for anyone that stops trying and let's children have their way without consequences and for those that assert dominance by taking away all choice of freedom.

Remember, consistency tempered with caring and love is critical. The youngster should understand that you do care about them. However, they need to recognize and acknowledge that they are not in a position to question their independence or make demands.

In the beginning, this will probably be hard. Still, if you keep on reflecting on it with decent patience, then you're going to be surprised with the numerous constructive outcomes. Remember, in the start, even if you are more lenient the child might feel like they have no room to breathe and complain to their parents and in that case you need to be patient as well.

You should not then go and provide explanations to the parents. Although, the parents will be curious and ask you about results and about their child's progress. You need to steer clear of unneeded grievance, and continuously work to better the child's perception and understanding while the need to coerce the child persists. Do not have a grudge and more importantly do not let the child hold a grudge. Children are inherently pliable, so, if you portray love while disciplining, they'll acknowledge it easily.

In case you've had a very difficult day with a youngster, talk to the parents of the child to explore possibilities of progress so that the child finds you soothing. Assessing your posture and trying to appear loving and act more caring to gain proximity to the child should be your strategy. Never be defensive and maintain tranquil and always keep a soft caring smile on your face.

Finally, I want to remind you that the only way our decent environment will work is if the educator and child work together after forming a connection.

Maybe it's a toy or a bicycle or a play-time activity that takes your child's attention. The independence authorized by the Montessori philosophy promotes the atmosphere, which causes all this to happen by natural means. Dr Montessori gave us the exact formula to establish this system but of course, for this to work, all the measures of this formula must be adopted. This is applicable in every region of lifestyle; a formulation isn't excellent if any other way is required.

Chapter 4: How to Discipline Toddlers?

The toddler's creed is, "If I want it, then it is mine. If I let you have it, and I change my mind, it is mine again. If it is mine, nobody can get it. If you build just like mine, it's mine. If we build something together, it is mine."

This is how toddlers think and feel. They believe the world revolves around them after watching how parents and other adults feed, fuss, and please them always. This is the period where parents need to become more efficient in teaching their children to adopt acceptable behavior and ethical values. Discipline is the cornerstone that will train your child to be responsible and become an asset to society.

What are toddlers?

Toddlerhood is from 1 to 3 years old (12 to 36 months). But there is no absolute definition of the limit of toddlerhood. Some say that the toddler age ends when the child is ready to enter preschool.

During this stage, toddlers display growth and developmental milestones in interrelated areas such as:

Physical & Motor

This refers to the increase in size and height, movement, and use of gross and fine motor skills.

Gross motor – the ability of the toddler to control their large muscles like arms and legs for walking, climbing, jumping and running

Fine motor – the ability to manipulate objects, draw, and feed themself using the small muscles of the hands and fingers

Social & Emotional

It includes the ability of the child to interact through playing games, fantasy play, taking turns, and how they identify their feelings and responds to others' emotions. It involves learning to adjust to the acceptable norms of the community while developing a sense of self and gaining independence.

Cognitive

This pertains to the child's capacity to understand abstract concepts and learn new skills. It is associated with intellectual capabilities, which include reasoning, thinking, knowledge acquisition, and the ability to process various information.

Communication

It encompasses language acquisition and verbal skills. It includes the ability to hear, interpret, and receive information. It also involves their ability to learn and understand language and using it to express themself.

As a parent, it's vital to remember that each child develops and grows at their unique pace, which is generally within the context of "normal development." If you think your child lagging in development, talking to their pediatrician will help you identify developmental delays that may require early interventions like speech, physical, or other therapies that helps them 'catch up' with peers.

At age 1 (12 months), toddler displays physical changes and can do the following skills:

1-4 Months

Physical & Motor Skills

Grows taller and heavier compared to birth weight and height.

The head circumference is equal to their chest.

Has 1-8 teeth.

Walks alone or with help.

Pulls themself to stand.

Sit down without any help.

Has a pincer grasp.

Turns book pages by flipping many pages.

Bangs blocks together.

Follows fast-moving objects.

Play ball by tossing or rolling it.

Cognitive Skills

Connects names with the objects.

Understands that objects exist, even if they aren't visible.

Social & Emotional Skills

Begins to develop an attachment to objects like toys.

Becomes mischievous and explores toys in new ways.

Enjoys simple games like peek-a-boo.

Starts to experience separation anxiety and becomes clingy when one or both parents leave.

Communication Skills

Understands some words and simple commands.

Responds when someone calls their name.

Responds to various sounds.

Can say one or more words like mama, papa, or dada.

Imitates animal sounds.

At age 2 (24 months), the typical toddler manifests:

Physical & Motor Skills.

Height is about 80 to 82 centimeters.

Weight is between 11 to 13 kilograms.

Has 12 temporary teeth.

Can walk up and down the stairs while holding on to the rail.

Develops total control of holding the spoon and feeds themselves.

Builds five cube towers successfully.

Becomes ready for toilet training.

Runs, throws, and kicks.

Likes to dress or undress themselves.

Copies circles and lines.

Holds crayon and pencil.

4-6 Months

Cognitive Skills

Learns to sort out toys or search for hidden objects.

Experiments to solve a problem.

Makes stories or creates games to play.

Sorts out color and shape.

Understands and follows more complicated instructions.

Understands simple acts like pushing buttons or turning on/off the lights.

Social & Emotional Skills

Imitates social behavior like feeding a doll or hugging a teddy bear.

Shows independence and starts to say "No" or throws a tantrum.

Displays attachment and separation anxiety.

Manifests self-recognition ability.

Begins to manifest tantrums when they are upset, tired, frustrated, or hungry.

Communication Skills

Can speak up to 50 words and continues to learn new ones.

Speaks in longer sentences, up to 4 words.

At age 3 (36 months), the toddler already mastered some of their newfound skills.

6-12 Months

Physical & Motor Skills

Grows in height and weight.

Can dress themselves.

Increased dexterity to solve puzzles and small objects.

Advanced climbing and mobility skills.

Draws and scribbles pictures, then telling you the story of their drawings.

Learns to peddle a bike.

Cognitive Skills

Plays with their toys in imaginative and creative ways.

Easily learns the people's names, places, and new words.

Builds structures using blocks.

Figures out how toys operate.

Plays make-believe games.

Social & Emotional Skills

Becomes more independent.

Anticipates routines.

Attempts to sing along with some songs.

Toilet learning continues.

Enjoys playing different games.

Picks their own entertainment and clothes.

Knows the difference between girls and boys.

Forms their own peer relationships.

Begins to navigate cooperation and sharing.

Communication Skills

Speaks in sentences.

With increasing vocabulary, they enjoy carrying on simple conversations.

Understands and follows 3 or more steps-direction.

Begins to understand more complicated concepts like below, inside, outside, and more.

The developmental timeline of toddlers varies from child-to-child. Some children show rapid development, while others display gradual changes. Nevertheless, they share similar patterns of skills development. They follow no rules and do things spontaneously, frequently changing toys, imitating others, and practicing make-believe play. They have a short attention span and enjoy throwing/retrieving objects.

They also learn to express themselves and display more emotions. They recognize colors, alphabets, and shapes. Children enjoy rhymes, songs, and games. Memorization comes easy for them because during the toddler stage because children are like sponges, soaking up everything that they see, hear, feel, and experience.

Significant Learning Milestones

Play (Parallel Play)

A parallel play is when children play adjacent to each other, each playing alone, but showing interest in what other children are doing. Play for toddlers is work. It helps them develop motor skills, sharpen skills (problem-solving, creativity, or critical thinking), and learn vital concepts (numbers, colors, or shapes). They are naturally curious, so make use of this phase to provide fun and educational activities that support their cognitive development and promote fine and gross motor skills.

Squatting

One and two-year-old toddlers usually play in a squatting position, with their feet wide apart and the bottoms not touching the floor. They squat instinctively from the standing position whenever they like to play or get something.

Potty Training

The toddler age is the perfect time to train your child proper toilet etiquette. Though, it is essential to determine if they are psychologically and physiologically ready. Physiological preparedness is the child's ability to perform necessary tasks such as sitting upright, controlling the urethral and anal sphincter, and walking. Psychological readiness refers to their ability to understand and follow directions and motivation to undergo toilet training.

Potty-training is one of the huge milestones for toddlers and a great challenge for parents. Keep in mind that your child needs to reach developmental milestones first and be interested in potty-training to make it a pleasant experience. Pushing a toddler too soon is not advisable because it can backfire and gives them trauma.

Language

Another exciting milestone that parents look forward to is hearing their children talk. Typically, the toddler utters their first word around 12 months and continues to build up vocabulary until 18 months. Beyond this age, their language rapidly increases and learns 7-9 words every day by mimicking people around them. At 21 months, your toddler starts to incorporate phrases into their vocabulary like "I go," "me play," or "mommy give." Moreover, they tend to engage in crib talk or monologue before sleeping.

Self-Awareness

Expect your toddler to begin recognizing themself as a separate person with abilities to think and act differently, including the feelings of pride and embarrassment.

Major Factors that Encourage Optimum Development of Toddlers

Food & Nutrition

At this stage, you can begin feeding your child with nutritious and well-balanced solid food. It is the ideal time to help them build healthy eating habits and introduce new foods. Toddlers need adequate nutrients, vitamins, and minerals to promote rapid growth and development at this stage. They need three meals and 1-2 snacks every day, which comprise whole grains, meat, vegetables, and fruits. Milk is also essential. A daily diet that lacks enough protein, fats, or carbs or has too much sugar that inhibits physical growth and brain development, along with issues of tooth decay and the risk of child obesity.

Take note that during this stage, some toddlers become picky eaters, so it's up to parents to become creative when introducing new foods to their kids. It is necessary to ensure that they get enough nutrients and plenty of calories. According to the American Academy of Pediatrics, a good measure of toddler portion size is about a quarter of the adult portion size. To handle food refusals and mealtime meltdowns, allow your kid more independence. Toddlers learn by mimicking their parents, so set a good example.

Sleep

Toddlers typically sleep 8-12 hours at night and take 1-2 naps during the day. Sleep is the fundamental requirement for the optimum growth and development of the child. It directly impacts the development of the brain. Lack of sleep makes children cranky, unpleasant, and prone to temper tantrums. It's important to stick to a routine that includes early bedtime and plenty of naps to prevent undesirable behaviors.

Safe Environment

A safe home and safe community are paramount to the child's social development and emotional health. It is vital to provide your child a healthy, caring, and secure environment that supports their optimum growth as they go through the toddler stage.

The risk factors that may cause developmental delays include poverty, violence in the home, the mother suffering from depression, drug use/abuse, and parent's mental health issues. Children whose parents are both working and spend a lot of waking hours with a nanny may experience delays in some aspects of development.

Interaction & Play

Toddlers basically learn from interaction and play during this phase of their lives, hence the necessity for parents and caregivers to provide opportunities for them to create, play, and explore. It's beneficial to keep the interactions engaging, caring, and loving.

Keep your child active at least 30 minutes with an adult-led structured physical activity or at least 1 hour of free play or unstructured physical activity. This will help your toddler gain balance, coordination, and muscle control. they are building a foundation that prepares their body for more complicated tasks like kicking, jumping, or running. Moreover, by allowing your child's natural desire to do more and keep moving, you're helping them establish a pattern of activity that they will adopt throughout their childhood and up to their adult life.

Medical Issues

Medical concerns can impede the normal growth and development of children. Those with serious or chronic diseases may experience slow physical development, while children with sight/hearing impairment may develop an inferiority complex, and other issues that affect their social development.

With prematurely born kids, it is necessary to adjust your child's developmental timeline and your expected milestones. Some toddlers may require physical, speech, or occupational therapy if there is an extreme delay in developmental milestones.

Why is it difficult to discipline a toddler?

Seeing children manifesting the first signs of aggression is very unsettling for parents. When the tiny fists of the toddlers go flying, followed by loud wailing, this is the sign that you need to start the discipline.

The first thing you need to remember when challenged by the behavior of your child is the fact that their brain isn't capable of rational thinking. According to experts, aggression during this phase of development is common because the prefrontal cortex (PFC), the tiny portion of the brain's frontal lobe is under major development. It continues to grow until the age of 25. At age 1 to 3, the child does not remember the rules. they do not understand why they need to be nice, make themself safe, or empathize with others. Their understanding of logic and consequences is still raw.

The age of two is the most critical year, often called the "terrible two" because toddlers display sudden temper tantrums when bored, tired, hungry, frustrated, or upset. Tantrums usually start at 9-months old and continue until parents unlock the reasons and resolve the issues that trigger them. As a parent, it's essential to assess if the method that you're using can calm the situation or set off another tantrum episode.

You need to realize that your child is in the exploratory stage, and they are testing the boundaries by trying the methods of seeking attention to get what they want when they want it. Your toddler is starting to discover things and wants to do them themselves. They are driven by the desire to assert themself and thus try hard to communicate their likes and dislikes. They are developing their sense of self, and it frustrates them when they cannot do it right. And because they cannot express themself clearly, your toddler vents their disappointment through unruly behavior and tantrums. These acts are their response to the situation, the best strategies that they believe are right, and capable of doing.

During this phase, you need to be more patient, empathetic, and aware of their developmental stage, applying age-appropriate discipline or response to correct the behavior. Setting rules and expectations that are too advanced for their current age usually leads to frustration, stress, anger, and a broken connection. It is better to avoid all these negative things to happen because, basically, you only want to correct the behavior of your child. Sure, disciplining requires firmness and directed effort, but it can be fun and engaging for you and your kid when you find the right balance.

In a nutshell, the behavior of the toddler can be erratic and unpredictable that can sap your sanity. they can switch from shy to aggressive or independent to clingy. It's because they aren't born with the necessary social skills and still trying to cope up with new things around him. This is where you teach them how to act safely and appropriately, so they can handle situations even when you aren't around. Your task is to implant a "memory chip" that will remind them constantly to be a good citizen. Consider it like taming a wild horse, but without the need to break your child's happy spirit.

It's important to realize that at this young age, modifying behavior through discipline is a journey that brings learning experiences to your toddler and you as well. Remember that the seeds of discipline you implant now will blossom and help them continue in the right path of adulthood.

Effective Ways to Teach Your Toddler Self-Control

Play fun games and activities that teach them impulse-control and self-control such as Hide N' Seek, Simon Says, Freeze (stop dancing when the music stops), Counting objects and numbers, Drumming, or Motor Games

Set appropriate boundaries and consequences

"If you hit someone, you have to stay in your calm down area."

"If you throw your toy, I will take it away."

Frequently talk about feelings and emotions to help them develop their emotional intelligence.

Keep the communication lines open.

Be patient when teaching them. Keep in mind that their brain is still developing, making it difficult for them to assimilate rules and expectations, so don't assume that they will understand and follow them consistently.

Statistics

According to UNICEF, over 80% of your child's brain is developed when they reach the age of three, and about 75% of the meal they eats goes to develop the brain. Moreover, a 15-minute play can spark thousands of connections in your child's brain.

Other pertinent facts:

- Lack of proper nutrition during early childhood can stunt growth and development.
- Poor sanitation, undernutrition, and other risks linked to poverty can cause developmental delays.
- 300 million kids below 5 years old are exposed to societal violence.
- 250 million children under 5 years old in middle-and-low-income nations face the risk of not reaching their full development potential because of extreme poverty.
- About 70% of kids between 2-4 years old experience being yelled or screamed at due to the practice of violent discipline in many nations.
- Worldwide, children aged 2-4 years old are regularly subjected to violent discipline and corporal punishment by their caregivers.

Children commonly experience violent discipline at home during their early years. Many caregivers and parents use physical and psychological methods to punish misbehavior and teach kids acceptable behaviors, including self-control. In their defense, parents or caregivers that use punishment as a form of discipline say they don't intentionally want to harm the child. They resort to it when faced with frustration and anger.

The lack of knowledge regarding the long-term effects of punishment on children is also a contributing factor. Governments invest little in the relevant programs, allocating only a very low budget on pre-primary education and other concerns. Also, public awareness of the importance of the child's first years is also low, resulting in a slight demand for funding the programs and policies.

Data in the National Parent Survey of Zero to Three revealed that 56% of parents believe that before the age of 3, children can resist the urge to do something forbidden, while 36% believe that kids below 2 years old can control this urge. It also showed that 44% of parents think strong resistance to breaking the rules happened during age 3 and older, and 18% believe that children can resist when they turn 6 months. When it comes to tantrums, 42% of parents believe that toddlers display them age 2, and they can also control their bodies. About 24% of parents say that their kids display tantrums by age 1 and show the ability to control their emotions.

Here is the reality. Research shows that self-control begins to develop between the ages of 3-½ and 4 years old. It means that controlled behavior is still hard for toddlers during these ages and below. So, don't expect a lot from your children during this period, but you can begin teaching, helping, and training them on how to control their impulses.

Common scenarios:

- "Do not touch the remote."
- "Do not run in the house."
- "Do not step off the sidewalk."

All these are everyday occurrences that parents deal with. If you think it's easy for your child to refrain from doing them, you are wrong. Because no matter how many times you tell them, they always want to test the limits and break the rules. The culprit is the lack of self-control because their brain cortex that influences the impulses and emotions aren't yet developed, so your child always acts without considering the ramifications.

Spanking & Child Behavior

Data showed that children who were spanked severely or frequently during the childhood stage tend to distance themselves from parents and face the greatest risk for mental health issues like depression and anxiety, along with drug and alcohol abuse.

The 2002 meta-analysis of 27 studies revealed strong evidence that children who experienced regular spanking display increased aggression that can continue until adulthood. Furthermore, they may have a misconception that violence is the way to gain power or get what they want from others. The tendency to bully, abuse partner, and other acts to overpower another person is often associated with the violence that children experienced in their early years of existence.

Child Skills and Spanking

The studies conducted in the 1960s and 2009 revealed a common result-there was a direct correlation between corporal punishment and the slow cognitive development of children. The latter revealed that children who were not spanked gained cognitive skills faster than those who constantly experienced it.

In 2013, Mackenzie et al. made a study using the Fragile Families and Child Well-Being longitudinal birth cohort approach. The result showed that high-frequency of fathers' spanking led to lesser scores in vocabulary among 9-year-old children.

Meanwhile, the 2010 Margolin et al. study about the Violence Exposure in Multiple Interpersonal Domains revealed that exposure of children and youth in violence at home and communities affects their emotional, physical, and academic adjustment. Experiencing violence, even once contributed to about 86.4% parent-to-youth aggression, 50.5% community aggression, and 59.2% physical marital aggression.

In the 2015 survey of the Pew Research Center, parents with kids under 18 said that they rarely used spanking as a method of discipline-only 4% admitted that they often do it, 43% frequently took away the privileges (use of the electronic device or TV, going out with friends), 41% with children below 6 years old used "time-out" approach, and 22% resorted to yelling.

Researchers who studied 4 national surveys that span 23 years of data found out that in 1988, 46% of mothers from middle-class families claimed that they used spanking as a discipline strategy. By 2011, the number decreased to 21%. In contrast, data showed that from 41%, the number of mothers who put their toddlers in time-out increased to 81%.

Chapter 5: When is Discipline Necessary?

Children are fantastic. They have a natural curiosity, innocence, and energy which allows them to see the world in unique ways. Toddlers are at the very beginning of a wonderful journey; to them, the world is full of new and exciting experiences. Unfortunately, toddlers and even young children aren't aware of the dangers which exist in the world around them, so it's your responsibility as a parent to guide them and keep them safe.

Discipline simply means creating a set of rules and guidelines to help your child grow into a healthy and considerate adult. More importantly, discipline will ensure that your child does not run into the road, randomly hit strangers, or even throw food around in a restaurant. Good discipline will allow you to go out to a variety of places with your toddler and enjoy the experience.

Unfortunately, it is simply not possible to draw up a standard set of rules which will miraculously provide you with the perfectly behaved child. Every toddler is different, and the influences and pressures placed on them will vary according to the pressure on you and your approach to each issue. **The guidelines you must create and enforce will be constantly changing!**

Good discipline is established by reacting positively to any situation and providing a reason why a specific type of behavior is necessary. It is also beneficial for your toddler to understand that there are consequences for not behaving properly. Likewise, consequences must be relative to the issue and you must carry through with it when your toddler has continued to behave badly. If you can't enforce the consequence, then your child won't have any incentive to behave in a respectful manner or learn the difference between right and wrong. Even when it's difficult to see your child upset, you must be aware that you're thinking of their future and this is more significant than anything else.

Types of Discipline

It should now be obvious that there are several different approaches to disciplining your child. In fact, there isn't one specific type which has been proven "better," and many parents will find that they have a preferred method but use a little of each approach:

Positive parenting

This is one of the better-known approaches and is being proven to have positive effects. Oregon State University started a research project in 1984 with 206 boys which they felt were at risk of juvenile delinquency; the children met with the researchers ever year until their 33rd birthday. The research has shown that positive parenting can improve behavior and interactions between generations.

As its name suggests, this approach to parenting and discipline relies on being positive to your child as much as you can. As a parent, you'll seek to remain calm, regardless of the situation. In return, traditional punishments, such as removing love or toys, remain as the idea is that your child will respond to you because of the bond you have with them and because they want to.

Reward and Punishment

This approach to discipline involves you creating the rules by which you expect your child to abide by. If they don't behave according to these rules, then you simply remove an item from them for a set amount of time; this will usually be their favorite toy.

If you adopt this approach, you'll need to be consistent - once you have said you'll remove the item, then you must do so. Although, this can often lead to another issue. A toddler may begin to realize that this is a result of their behavior, yet this won't stop them from being upset and you'll then need to decide whether to comfort them or not.

Research suggests that this is the fundamental flaw with this type of parenting because most parents will not wish to remove a toy as it feels wrong. Unfortunately, if you say you're going to do something and then don't, you will have just taught your toddler that they can push it further the next time. Equally, if you do remove the item and then comfort your upset child, you will be effectively rewarding their bad behavior with comfort which can encourage them to repeat the bad behavior.

Reward and punishment are often referred to as "tough love." This is because it can be tough on the parent and your child.

Behavior Modification

There is a technique which involves ignoring naughty or disrespectful behavior. In contrast, praise and rewards are offered when your child does something right. If ignoring complaints or behavior does not stop the behavior, then a punishment would need to be awarded.

This approach focuses on consequences but will often overlap with the reward and punishment approach.

Emotional Discipline

Children are subject to the same range of emotional responses as adults. In many situations, they will be unsure of their feelings and how they should influence their approach to an issue. This type of discipline encourages your child to open up about their feelings. The belief is that understanding their emotions will allow them to learn how to deal with them and how to react positively in any situation.

Research suggests that there is merit in this approach. Children capable of dealing with emotions properly will generally be calmer like adults and adapt to a variety of situations.

Commanding

This is the old-fashioned approach to parenting and is based on the premise that children should be seen and not heard. Adopting this approach means that you expect your children to do exactly as they are told. If not, then you'll immediately dish out punishment with no specific reward for good behavior. Punishment can range from loss of toys to physical spanking.

This approach works more along the lines of fear than love. It isn't seen as an appropriate or effective long-term method, and many children who have been brought up this way will reach their teenage years and rebel against the strict rules. The result is a child which does all the things that you have taught them not to. In addition, in many cases, the relationship between parent and child is, at best strained; more likely, it's simply non-existent.

Merits of Positive Parenting

Discipline is the means by which you guide your toddler into becoming a well-rounded child and subsequently, a positive adult. It's generally accepted that this is the best method for guiding your toddler into adulthood whilst retaining a strong bond between you and them.

There are several merits associated with this approach:

Recognizing feelings

Your toddler is surprisingly aware of what is happening around them. If they see from a young age that you are sad when they don't follow your guidelines, they will resist doing these things. This is because they will want to keep you happy which is a natural desire in children.

By starting this at toddler age, you will enable your child to understand how their actions affect others and take this into consideration before they act.

Emotions

Just as your toddler will learn your feelings and how to consider others before they act, they will also react to a positive parenting approach by feeling good about themselves. This is inevitable. A toddler will see that you're happy when they respond in a certain way, which will generate additional positive attention for them, and they will quickly realize that they like the feeling. In turn, you can encourage them to feel good when they achieve something.

In contrast, if you adopt a punishment-based system, you will generally find that your child is afraid to make a decision or speak up because they don't want to incur the consequences of a bad decision. This will stunt their emotional growth.

Personality Development

It's highly likely that you enjoy being praised. After all, everyone likes to be recognized for what they do as praise inspires you to try again and achieve even greater things. The same is true when you apply a positive parenting approach to your toddler. Although young, they will quickly recognize the benefits and satisfaction of having reached for something and achieving it.

Although your child is just a toddler, this can be one of the best times to start this approach. After all, they will have just started walking and are ready to try a host of new things!

Integration

Whilst you don't need to raise a child that simply follows the herd, you do want your child to be aware of how their actions affect others. This will allow them to develop the best approach to any issue whilst keeping most people happy. Only by adopting this approach in the adult world will they be able to achieve great success.

How to Implement Positive Parenting

Deciding to be a positive parent does not mean that it will always be easy to achieve! In fact, learning to be a positive parent can often mean saying "yes" to your toddler when you may have said "no." The inclination to be overly permissive is a downside of the positive parent approach, but this is usually only temporary as you work out how to be a positive parent and which approach works best for you.

The following guidelines should help you implement your positive parenting approach:

Know the Limits

Your toddler is just starting to get around on their own. As an adult, you'll be aware of a huge number of potential issues, most of which will revolve around how your toddler can hurt themselves. You can choose to wrap your child in cotton wool, but they will never learn what they can achieve and may never push the boundaries.

You can also choose to say "no" all the time to prevent them from doing anything dangerous. Unfortunately, despite having their best interests in mind, saying "no" all the time will simply leave your toddler switched off. In addition, if you say "no," and they do it anyway, then you'll need to follow through with your "punishment." It is highly unlikely that you'll have the time or the energy to follow through on all the incidents as your toddler will, after all, be keen on pushing their limits.

A better approach is to set your own limits. You must decide which actions are fundamentally likely to be dangerous or affect their long-term growth. Knowing that they could fall over and hit their head on the coffee table is not a good enough reason to say "no" to them walking! You must look at every situation and decide if it's likely to be an issue in the future, in which case, a "no" is a worthwhile response; just ensure that it's backed up with solid reasons. Even a toddler can understand the reason for your actions if you demonstrate it.

Consistency

Children like to think they are older than they are. But in reality, they aren't in a rush to be making their own decisions; they simply want reassurance that you're there to keep them safe. The best way to reassure them of this and allow them to respect your judgment and decisions is to be consistent.

Again, you should only deal with the issues that are of a fundamentally significant nature. But, once you have decided that there is a right and a wrong regarding a specific action, then you must be consistent. Toddlers will quickly learn when they shouldn't be doing something, but if you keep changing the rules, they will become confused and are likely to continue the antagonizing action.

Stay Calm!

After a long day, a toddler that will not do as they are told can be the final straw. This is when it can be most difficult to stay calm and when it's the most important time to do so.

Connectivity

Positive parenting revolves around connecting with your toddler. If they have misbehaved, you must connect with them before you deal with their actions. This can be as simple as picking them up or making eye contact with them.

Connecting assures them of your love, making it easier to communicate with them and explain why their actions were wrong. You can then ask or talk to them about the issue and deal with it.

Acknowledge Them

Once your toddler has crossed a boundary, you'll need to ensure they know it's unacceptable behavior. Connecting with them reassures them but acknowledging them helps to gain their cooperation.

As an adult, you generally respond better to praise and the feeling that your point of view has been understood. A toddler may struggle to express their viewpoint, but if you express it for them and ask them to confirm if, you're giving them the opportunity to be understood. In turn, this will make them want to accept the limits you are imposing simply because you have emphasized with them.

Stepping In

You must decide when it is appropriate to step in. In general, this can be decided before most incidents. For example, if your toddler hits someone, you must intervene immediately. However, if they are arguing with another toddler, it can be acceptable to watch and see how they deal with the situation. You will, of course, need to be ready to step in!

Build Your Relationship

The bond between you and your toddler is essential, and you should take every opportunity you can to strengthen this. Instead of waiting for them to do something good and positively encouraging them, you can spend time with them and create the situations that gives way to encouraging and stimulating comments.

But, perhaps most importantly, you need to remember the importance of simply spending time with them without judging their actions. This will improve your bond and ensure they want to please you, making your boundaries much easier to enforce.

It's also worth noting that if you're going to use consequences as a method of teaching, then you must be prepared to avoid intervening. Every time you intervene, the consequence will be transferred into a punishment inflicted by you and not simply a result of their actions. For a consequence to be effective, your child must complete the action and learn the lesson the hard way; this can be difficult to watch, but it's a very effective way of teaching.

Chapter 6: Encouraging Good Toddler Behavior

One of the most effective ways to encourage positive behavior in children is through praise. Children seek love and recognition for their efforts and progress. Praise increases children's self-confidence and motivation by making them feel happy. It's beneficial to give them confidence in their abilities and to show them that they feel

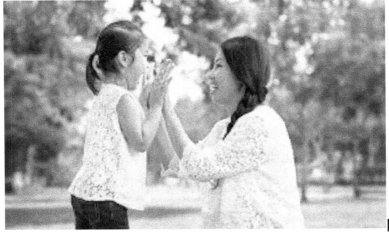

proud when they behave correctly, thereby encouraging good behavior. Here are some highly effective tips to help encourage positive behavior.

Encourage Effort

Use praise to encourage effort and to enhance the progress of your child. A child who can use the bathroom alone for the first time or perform a task that they were not able to do before deserves recognition. In this way, it is encouraging the child's development and autonomy.

Reinforce Attitudes

Enjoy instilling some values that you consider fundamental, important, and positive. By praising and reinforcing attitudes, you help to develop social skills that will make relationships easier in the future.

Praise the Effort, Regardless of the Result

The effort must be praised even if the goal is not fully achieved. If your child did not receive an excellent grade, but studied and worked for this to be possible, it's significant to recognize him. Praise is key to staying motivated and, hence improving your bottom line.

Praise Good Behavior

It's important to praise good behavior; don't save compliments only for great achievements. Small behavior improvements should also be valued. If we only pay attention at times where behavior needs work, children will feel inclined to do wrong.

Approve or Disregard Attitudes and Not the Child

As much as you consider your child to be very handsome, intelligent, etc., avoid telling them this often. This type of label turns out to be as harmful as the opposite ("you're dumb," "you're bad," etc.). Try to mark your approval or disapproval regarding attitudes, not the child.

Value the Achievements of the Family

It is significant to value the achievements and efforts of the family. If a child has accomplished something, it's important to praise them, as well, any achievements of the family members. It is beneficial to recognize the effort of all the elements and celebrate the achievements in the family.

Rewards

You can also choose to reward your child, such as a gift, a trip to the movies, or candy if you want to reinforce an attitude. But don't make it a routine because this can lead to only good behavior when rewarded. Most behavior should be rewarded only by praise. Also, you may be tempted to use the allowance as a reward. We don't recommend it. Never use the allowance to "buy" your child.

Rewarding the child for good behavior teaches them to understand that there is a direct link between action and consequence.

Remember that as a parent you are a role model for your children. It's essential that you be a good role model by providing them with appropriate rules and standards to follow. Consistency is the key. Children learn by observing others, and they will learn these qualities. With a little persuasion and positive reinforcement, you can teach, encourage, and create positive behavior in children.

How to Stimulate Good Behavior in Children?

Stimulating good behavior in children is one of the best ways to impose limits, without having to apply punishments constantly. The only problem is how to do that. In most cases, our little ones tested our limits and seem to do anything not to obey.

Be the Example

Being an example is the most effective way we need to teach our children anything - both good and bad. When it comes to encouraging good behavior in children, it is no different. Here are a few examples of what you can do for your child to learn.

Catch your child's attention when you split snacks with your husband or when you have to wait in the bank queue, pointing out that adults also have to share and wait too.

Realize the Good Behavior

If you are like any parent in the world when your child is behaving well, you leave them playing alone and take advantage of the time to do anything you may need to. But when your child is behaving badly, you direct all your attention to them to resolve the situation. Your attention is what kids most want, so to get this attention sometimes children will behave badly. The best way to encourage good behavior in children is to pay attention when they are behaving well and to take your attention from them when they are behaving badly. This is completely counter-intuitive for us and can be a difficult habit to cultivate. But once you get used to it, it will become easier and easier.

A great way to do this is to play with your child when they are quiet in their corner and praise them when they obey you the first time you speak.

Understand the Stage of Development

This tip is easy to understand. Each child has a behavior; though, you cannot require a child of three to act as the same as a child that is ten. That is, do not try to go to a three-hour lunch with your little boy hoping they will be quiet for the whole lunch. Do not expect a two-year-old child to stop stuffing everything in their mouth. Each age has a phase, and it is no use wanting to demand different behavior from a child.

Have Appropriate Expectations

This is a continuation of the above tip. Parents have high expectations. This is not wrong when expectations are possible. For example, don't expect a tired child to behave well, or a one-month-old baby to sleep through the night.

Create Structure and Routine

A child with a structured routine tends to behave better. They already know what to expect and are used to it. A child with a routine feels safe and thus lives more calmly. A child without a routine has a sense of insecurity that will disrupt much in the time to educate and encourage good behavior.

Uses Disciplinary Strategies

Rather than humiliating or beating children, there are positive disciplinary strategies that teach them the right things, set boundaries, and encourage good behavior in children. Some of these are: give options, put somewhere to think, talk, give affection and a system of rewards (reward can be a simple compliment, it does not have to be gifts or food).

Understand That the Bad Behavior Worked So Far

If throwing tantrums and disobeying worked for them to get your attention so far, changing this behavior will take time. They will have to understand that you will no longer pay attention to them when they behave badly, but when they behave well.

Instilling good behavior practices in young children is a must for any responsible parent, but sometimes it can also be quite complicated and laborious. Although, beginning to instill this type of behavior as early as possible will help build a good foundation for the child's behavior and attitudes in the future. It's necessary to be aware that in the first years of life the children are like "sponges" and results will be better if you begin to show them early and direct them to appropriate behaviors of life in society.

More ideas to help parents with the task of encouraging good **behavior in their children**

Models to Follow

Children tend to mirror the behaviors of parents and those with whom they coexist more closely. So, be careful about your behaviors and language when the child is around to avoid misunderstanding ideas and misconceptions about how you should behave towards others. This includes talking properly and behaving politely to both your partner and family, as well as to the child. Try to avoid loud, unstructured arguments when the child is around. We do not mean you can't disagree with your spouse, because the child must also be aware that these exist. But try to have the arguments always controlled and civil around children.

Be Firm

Parents should be affectionate, but still adamant about instilling discipline in their children. It is important that the child knows how to respect their parents, even when they do not have what they want. Understanding when to say "no" at the right times is a significant step in your education.

Positive Body Language

Your body language has a huge impact when you are trying to instill a certain behavior in children. Given the height of the child, a parent standing while correcting the errors and applying discipline is often viewed as authoritative. It is advisable to place yourself at the same level as the child's eyes. Sit next to the child while talking to them and always maintain eye contact.

Establishing Limits

It is fundamental to establish limits, rules, and consequences for unwanted behavior. Increase limits on children to be able to distinguish right from wrong. They need to know what is not acceptable and clear reasons that make it wrong so that there is no doubt in the child's mind about the behavior to adopt.

You started tracking your child's progress long before they left the warmth of your belly: in the tenth week, the heart began beating; on the 24th week, their hearing developed and listened to your voice; in the 30th week, they began to prepare for childbirth. Now that they are in your arms, you're still eager to keep up with all the signs of your little one's development and worries that they might be left behind. Nonsense! Excessive worry won't help at all, so take your foot off the accelerator and enjoy each phase. Your child will realize all the fundamental achievements of maturity. They will learn to walk, talk, potty, and when you least expect it, they'll be riding a bicycle alone (and no training wheels!). They will do all this in time.

Stop taking developmental milestones so seriously. For example, your 7-month-old son will be able to sit alone and at age 3 will be able to ride a tricycle. Consider what is expected for each age just for reference. The best thing to do is to set aside the checklist of the abilities your child needs to develop and play together a lot. There is no better way to connect with and develop your child than through playtime.

To help you even further in realizing the goals mentioned above or processes, I would like to mention some tips here that stimulate a child's intellectual, motor, social, and emotional development:

Rainbow

The baby starts noticing colors at around 3 months of age when the vision is no longer so blurry. That is why, at this age, the idea is to stimulate with strong colors, which can be in toys or mobile in the crib. Babies also love contrast: you can see that stripes aren't missing in children's toys. At about a year and a half, your child will notice the difference between one color and another, even if they do not know the color's name. So, start saying: "Let's play with that blue ball" or "Take the red tomato from the salad." This way colors become part of their day to day life.

Books

The role of parents is fundamental for children to learn to love reading and to make books a pleasure, rather than an obligation. According to the latest edition of the Portraits of Reading survey in Brazil, for 43% of readers, the mother was the main influence for developing the desire for reading, and for 17%, the father was the one who played the role. From the third month of your child's life, you can use plastic books in the bath. From the sixth, when the baby can already carry objects to the mouth with their hands, leave cloth books in the cradle - in addition to being able to bite them, they won't be able to rip the pages! At all ages, talk about the cover, the pictures, the colors and let the child turn the pages.

Memory

Memory is a form of storing knowledge and must be permeated by a context. Start by helping your child memorize words by showing a represented object. If you're walking on the street and crossing a bicycle, point and say, "Look, son, a bicycle." This is how they will build associations. From the first year, they will say a few words and try to repeat the names of what you show. But it is from the age of 2 that the ability to retain information increases.

Creating

Create characters and a dream of fantastic worlds. All of this is cardinal in developing the creativity of little ones; it also contributes to problem-solving. To make the narrative more exciting, how about testing the improvisational ability of the two of you? Separate figures from objects, landscapes, colors, foods, and animals – they can be drawn or cut from magazines. While one narrates, the other can select images that portray elements that should be included in the narrative. The challenge is to be able to fit them together so that the narrative continues to make sense. By age 7, as the child is already literate, you can help them record your adventures in small booklets.

Always Ask

When picking up your child from school, you say, "How was your day?" And they say, "Cool." It was not exactly what you wanted to hear, right? To avoid generic responses, develop the questions so that the child needs to express what they think and justify their response. Ask: "What did you enjoy most today?" And they will be forced to develop more elaborate reasoning, requiring them to work linguistic and logical skills. At 3 years old, they can already relate experiences they went through and say whether those were good or bad. At 4, you can ask for details, descriptions, and names of colleagues who were with him.

Blessed Doubt

"Why does a dog not eat pizza?" "Was Grandma Ever a Child?" Although child questioning can make adults uncomfortable or embarrassed, these are essential for understanding the child's world. It is the process of distinguishing between real and imaginary (which occurs around the age of 4) and the construction of relations between known elements. That's why the "why questions" are paramount in the child's development process. Even if you don't know how to respond to everything your child asks, show that their or their them concern is relevant, and recognize when you don't know the answer.

Play, Clean, Play

As your child plays, insist that they engage in one game at a time, to build concentration. "Do you not want to play bowling anymore?" From age 2, your child can help clean up the toy they were using, before picking up a new one, so they also develop the sense of organization.

Belly-Down

Your child begins to strengthen the body between the first and the sixth month. Because thick motor development (involving the activities of large muscles such as sitting and walking) occurs in the head to toe direction, the first step is to strengthen the neck muscles. Beginning the first month, give your child at least two periods a day supported belly downtime on a flat and firm surface. In this way, the baby can lean securely and lift their head. At 6 months, they will start to sit alone. Arrange several cushions around them to help them get stronger.

Clap, Clap, Tum, Tum

One of the best ways to develop motor coordination is to teach rhythm to your child. To do this, just use your hands. From the seventh month, clap with them to the sounds of your favorite songs, interspersing slow songs with other accelerated songs, so they can see the difference. You'll see that your baby will be able to smack their little hands.

Everything Fits

From the age of 7 months, the baby begins to hold objects; in about a year and a half, they will begin to put pieces together. Besides being a good exercise for coordination, the child will learn which part will fit within the other. For your child to enjoy and learn from this, they can play with pots and plastic mugs while you prepare lunch. From the age of two and a half, also offer small puzzles (about six pieces).

Step by Step

Climbing stairs is a great exercise to develop agility and coarse motor coordination, as well as assisting to strengthen muscles. At 1 year of age, the child can already perform the activity, but only by placing both feet on the same step, one at a time. With growth, they will gain strength and balance until by age 3, they will probably rise by placing one foot on each step alternately. Even at this stage, it's important that they be accompanied by an adult to avoid accidents.

Bonding & Trust

Establishing relationships of trust is significant for the development of the child. The first people they do it with are the parents. For this, one factor is essential: never lie. If the child goes to the doctor to take a vaccine, don't even think about saying that you're just going for a walk. If they ask if the injection will hurt, be honest and say it will, yes, but it will pass. The experts are all in agreement: explain everything. Tell them he's going to get wet, it's going to hurt, he's going to be cold, so they know what to expect and learns to trust what you say.

Congratulate your child when they are good at something, encouraging them to continue. If scolding is necessary, pay close attention to how to do it. Saying "what you did was naughty" is quite different from saying "you are naughty!" Don't let the child think that the criticized trait is part of their personality, so they won't incorporate this trait into their self-image.

Chapter 7: The Listening Process

To understand your listening behavior's, and to increase your active listening skills, you're going to learn about the listening process. Don't be afraid! A little theory will help you to understand listening and give you the knowledge to apply it to your interactions.

There are several stages involved in the process of listening. Despite being distinct phases, they happen almost simultaneously as you look. They are, in brief, as follows:

Receiving-This is the physical function of hearing, where you receive the actual sound as vibrations in your ear, transmitted to your brain. As well as audio, any visual cues such as body language and eye contact will also picked up on.

Attending-When the message has received, i.e. physically picked up on by your senses and carried to your brain, it must then participate. At this stage, it's your job to pay attention to the message by holding it firmly in the short-term memory (Baddley & Hitch, 1974). The more attention you pay to the signals of the speaker at this stage, the more likely you are of taking in what communicated. It's essential in active listening to pay close attention to the speaker because without doing so, and it's impossible to interpret and respond to what is said.

Perceiving-As the amount of attention you pay to the speaker, your perceptions are also a part of the listening process. This may sound unusual at first, but your background, experiences, beliefs, and your state of mind at the time, will all affect the message that you eventually receive. In short, you hear what you want to hear, or sometimes what you expect to hear. This is one of the reasons why two people may listen to a different message from the same speaker; their perceptual filters have screened out or amplified different parts of the word.

You must have a perceptual filter. There are so many potential incoming signals in the world that it would simply blow your mind to take them all in. This can even be seen in essential functions like crossing the road, where you'll notice (if you try) that you'll be more attuned to the noise of cars, speed and distance, and to move in that moment. You may also blank out a lot of what else is around until you have made it to the other side.

Interpreting-So far on the journey, you have picked up the speaker's communication with your senses, which have carried it to the brain. You have held your attention on it for long enough that you have remembered it, and your perceptions have meanwhile done a great job of filtering out what is not needed, or what is in too severe a conflict with your conceptual outlook. Now, communication will be processed for meaning.

Your brain does this by attempting to fit the message into the correct linguistic categories, where it can discern meaning according to your previous experiences, thoughts and beliefs, and long-term memory. Linguistic groups are a technical term for how we break down how common people speak into categories and if needed analyze them.

In layman's terms, this means that you interpret, and possibly an analysis of what has been said. You decide yourself at this point what understanding you get from the speaker's message, and what the meaning is. Often the original meaning can be distorted and can even end up completely different to what it meant initially.

One of the main aims of active listening is that it seeks to understand what was meant by the speaker, rather than assuming our interpretation is correct.

Responding-The final stage of the listening process is the response. Internally, you are moving the message from short term to long term memory in case you need to retrieve it at a later point. The external response is given in the form of feedback, which may be an agreement, a reiteration or paraphrase, or a question regarding the message. The answer is an essential part of listening. Research by Leavitt and Mueller (1968) showed that the listener and speaker both gain confidence that the message has been understood and both experience a high degree of satisfaction in conversation when feedback is given. This is something that active listening places a lot of emphasis on and will be covered in more detail later on in the book. A response can go beyond feedback and can represent a transition between listening and speaking.

Chinese Whispers

You may be a little bogged down after that, but you must be familiar with the listening process; it provides a solid foundation for everything that is to come. For now, you can consider the above method of listening in the context of a game of Chinese whispers.

If you aren't familiar with the game, Chinese whispers played in a group, who sit on a circle. Someone picked to start the game, by coming up with a message to pass on to the person next to them. They think of a word and whisper it in the next person's ear, and it passed all the way around. The last person in the circle shouts the message out loud, and the original speaker reveals the original message. Then everyone laughs at how much the word has changed and tries to work out where" the distortions occurred.

So, where do the distortions occur" How did "My uncle packed sandwiches for all of us to take to the beach," become "Try walking up this way to get to get to the sweets."?

Well, the distortions could occur at any point during the communication, and the more people the message goes around, the more distorted it is likely to become.

It could be a lack of attention and only part of the message received by someone. It could be that the message has been screened out by bias or misinterpreted by the impressions of someone. If the idea is emotionally charged or opinionated, then this is even more likely.

If you have not played this game yet, then consider getting it together to see how flawed our listening can be, even when the message is simple.

Why Is It Helpful to Understand This Process?

It's easy to see from studying the listening process described above that listening is a somewhat complicated process that involving multiple aspects. Instead of merely labeling yourself as a "bad listener," you can begin to understand what you can improve upon, or what stage of the listening process might be causing you to miss what is going on in the communication.

Do you pay enough attention to what is said? Is there a reason for you not doing? Are there too many actions in the room? Maybe you block out the real message because you don't want to hear it; it could be your perceptual filter which causes you to cross wires with your loved ones. You could be misinterpreting the message that your friend is conveying. You may not be providing enough feedback for the speaker, who is relying on your response to engage in the conversation.

By understanding the whole process of listening, you can begin to see it differently. You can start to understand it.

A Positive Listening Attitude

Just in case your mind has been blown by the theory covered so far, you'll be glad to know the tension will be momentarily released, and some simple advice offered to all of you. All the steps of the process above can easily enhance with a positive listening attitude.

A positive listening attitude is to be interested in what is said. It varies across the conversation, and natural interest rises and falls depending on your concern for the message at hand. But being genuinely interested in what people have to say, and being open-minded towards new perspectives, helps you to function smoothly as a listener. Where your loved ones are concerned, you should always be interested.

Seeing listening as an active role in interaction also helps to cultivate this attitude. As a listener, it is your job to facilitate conversation. Please begin to see listening for the shining grace that is a valuable skill, and it helps people to feel relaxed in their relationships with you.

Start to enjoy listening; be positive open-minded.

"What Is an Active Listener?"

You may have seen the words "active listener" mentioned several times in this book already; you may have also seen it mentioned elsewhere.

In Western culture, we often listen in a somewhat passive way; we wait our turn while the other person speaks. We keep quiet out of respect for their message. Often, we are waiting for our turn again.

The active listener is engaged. They are as much a part of the conversation as the speaker because they see themselves as being partially responsible for the communication. They have a positive attitude towards listening; they are consciously working out what the message means, what angle the speaker is approaching from, and what their response may be. An active listener gives full attention to the conversation and is interested in what is said, why it is said, and how the speaker can be encouraged.

Chapter 8: Discipline Vs. Punishment

It must be noted that discipline and punishment are different. On the one hand, punishment has a punitive nature and does not change the behavior of a child. In many cases, punishment can even make the situation worse. The child only suffers and learns nothing. Unfortunately, punishment also tends to subject the child to humiliation, serious discomfort, anger, more frustrations, and anxiety, among others.

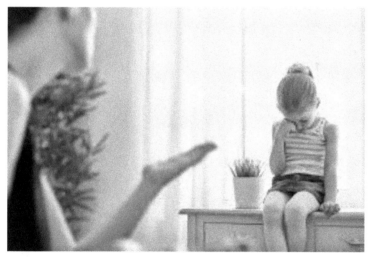

On the other hand, effective discipline is both safe and healthy for the child. Although punishments are also used in an effective discipline strategy, such punishments are mild and only play a part of the whole strategy. Last but not the least, punishment controls a child while discipline guides a child, allowing them to learn from their mistakes and grow beautifully.

Say No to Spanking

Although spanking can be traced back to ancient times to discipline a child, various studies today show that it isn't effective. Spanking can even make the situation worse. Spanking a toddler tends to make the child more aggressive, and it does not teach them the right conduct.

Spanking is based on pain. The theory behind it is that a person would not continue doing something that harms him. For example, if you touch a hot stove with your bare hands, you'll get hurt, remove your hands immediately, and would no longer dare to do the same thing again. Although this sounds logical enough, disciplining a child isn't as simple as avoiding getting burned by a hot stove. When you discipline a child, you not just tell the child what not to do but also what to do. Discipline teaches positive toddler behaviors, which lead them to take positive actions.

Another thing that makes spanking harmful is that the child tends to lose trust in their parents. Your toddler looks up to you for support, comfort, and care. If you become a source of pain to them, especially more frequently, then your child will step back and put a shield around themself. This naturally damages the parent-child relationship.

If you are a parent who is used to spanking your child probably because that was how you were "disciplined" when you were young, or maybe because you simply thought it was the best way to save from child from being a bad person, here are five ways that you can do to stop yourself from spanking your child and be a better parent.

Learn to Use Words

Use words instead of physical aggression. Control yourself and talk calmly without scolding and be sure to use words that your child can understand. Toddlers have a short attention span and cannot analyze things as well as adults, so keep your words short and simple. Since you communicate with words, you must also listen to your child. It should be a two-way conversation so that there will be understanding. It is also likely that there will be fewer problems if your child feels that you're listening to them. Just as you get exasperated when you feel that your child cannot understand what you are saying, your child also feels terrible when you do not listen to him.

Shift of Focus

Many times, all it takes is a shift of focus. Instead of focusing too much on the negative, focus on the positive behaviors. By giving all the time to positive things, there is no opportunity for the negative behaviors even to manifest themselves.

Let them Learn on their Own

As people always say, "Experience is the best teacher." This is also true for toddlers. There are times that you don't have to spank your child just for them to learn. By simply letting the normal flow of things to unfold by itself, your toddler can learn from their actions. For example, if they continue to play with their toy despite your warning roughly, the toy can soon break. This will teach your toddler a good lesson, which is more effective than simply spanking and hurting your child. But, of course, if there is a risk that is threatening to the life and well-being of your child, then you should intervene immediately and explain to your child the potential serious consequences.

Take a Timeout

Take a timeout except that this time, you should be the one who should take the timeout. Just before you lose your cool, give yourself a break. Step back for a minute and cool your temper. It is important to note that you should not face your toddler when you aren't calm and centered. Unfortunately, if you're in a public place and you cannot step back and leave your kid alone, the best thing you can do is to pray and think of happy thoughts.

Have the Realization that Spanking does not Help

Time and again, various studies show that spanking is not a good way to discipline a child. Spanking can only make things worse, and it does not make you a good parent. Hence, instead of spanking your child, think of more ways that are positive and constructive on how you can correct the wrong behavior.

Four Pillars of Effective Discipline

The most effective techniques to discipline a child are characterized by four factors, which make them not only effective but also safe and healthy for the child. Unlike punishment, the four pillars of effective discipline promote childhood learning and welfare.

It builds a positive parent-child relationship

Effective discipline should be supportive of the relationship between the parent and the child. Unlike punishments that are based on fear, effective discipline is based on understanding, love, and support. You should keep in mind that toddlers are very sensitive, and their early childhood relationships have a great influence on their brain development, as well as on their behavior. By building up a positive relationship with your toddler, they will not only learn the right conduct but also enjoy a strong bond of love and trust with you.

It is safe.

The safety of the child is of utmost importance. This is another reason why smart parent frown upon the use of punishments that involve bodily harm. Sometimes, the punishments can turn into cruelty and no longer serve the best interest of the child. Not to mention, many of such serious punishments are inflicted when the parent has already lost their patience and control of the situation.

It has reasonable expectations.

Discipline teaches the child the proper conduct. Thus, you should also consider the age and brain development of your child in making your expectations. Positive behaviors should be continuously enforced, while negative behaviors should be suppressed as early as possible. Be sure to take notice every time your child demonstrates good behavior, or at least try to do so.

It is composed of multiple techniques that are safe for the child.

Effective discipline is a system of techniques or strategies. A certain technique is used depending on the situation. And, again, this pillar highlights the importance of the child's safety. Every challenging behavior should be taken as a learning opportunity, which can allow the child to learn and grow. As a parent, you must be able to approach the problem directly in a calm manner.

Is it too late?

Some people think that it is too late to exercise discipline and that their toddlers can no longer change. It is worth noting that toddlers experience rapid changes. Change is part of being a toddler. Either you turn bad behavior into good behavior, or let the bad behavior get worse. Of course, as a loving parent, you only want what is best for your child. So, if you're one of the many who think that it might be too late to begin using some discipline, then it should be clear to you by now that it's never too late to do so. Scientifically speaking, it's best to help your child grow in a positive light while they are still a toddler. If they get to bring certain bad behavior up to their adulthood, they will be more difficult to correct.

What if it does not work?

Another common dilemma shared by most parents is what if nothing changes even if they try to discipline their child? There are certain points to consider. First, there are many techniques that you can use to discipline your child. Second, you won't know if it will work unless you take action to do so. Third, changing bad or inappropriate behavior takes time and effort. Fourth, toddlers usually have more than a single behavior that you should try to improve. By applying a form of effective discipline, you can at least help them change some of their bad behaviors. If you're lucky enough, you might put right all their inappropriate manners. Fifth, exercising discipline increases the chances that your child will grow as a good person. Sixth, change happens not only in toddlers but also in adults. Hence, there is no good reason to think that you cannot change your child's behavior. At the least, you can teach them some good manners. Last but not the least, it is your responsibility as a parent to do everything for your child, to make them grow the best way you can.

All kids need boundaries. Boundaries aren't only a great way to teach your toddler good behavior, but they also help them feel safe and secure. The tricky part about boundaries is setting and enforcing them. This becomes a little difficult, especially if you want to avoid bribing, threatening, or coercing your child to listen to you. You must be calm and set firm limits for your child. This is a simple exercise you must repeat time and again, without any inconsistencies. There are no timeouts when it comes to parenting - you're in it for the long haul.

Whenever your child is being rude or starts behaving in an unsafe manner, and you're about to burst, you'll experience powerful emotions. You are human too, and the way you handle your emotions in these situations sets the tone for future conversations. Your body shifts into a fight or flight mode when your fuse has gotten short, and your body is flooded with a steady stream of adrenaline and cortisol. These two chemicals prevent any form of rationalization that can take place in your brain. At this point, rationalization has effectively gone out of the window. Your ability to think is naturally hampered while your emotions run amok. Apart from this, your perception of the given situation is also skewed because of such powerful emotions you experience. The best way to regain control of the situation is by reminding yourself that parenting is not a sprint and is a marathon. If you don't want to harm the relationship you share with your toddler and at the same time want to set some limits or boundaries for him, then here are some steps you must follow.

Chapter 9: How Effective Communication Plays A Role in Toddler Discipline

Communication with your child represents an open door. The child will often initiate a conversation (sometimes it can be an open invitation for help), but the question is whether you will recognize this call for help, hear it, and answer it with an adequate response. If you invest in communication with your child, this becomes the foundation on which you build a lasting relationship.

Some of the fundamental laws of good communication with your child are:

Consider their age. You can already begin to explain the "great" secrets of life to your three-year-old child. It's surprising, but your toddler can understand how children are born, whether there is a God, what happens when someone dies, and similar things. Still, when you're talking to a child, the principle is always the same: tell the truth using words the child is already familiar with.

Communication is a two-way street when you share your everyday experiences with a child rather than expecting them just to talk to you. If you get a detailed answer to the question of how your toddler spent the day, the child deserves to receive a detailed answer to their question as well.

Share your personal opinions. You don't have to always keep things in confidence just because of the different levels of a child's thinking. On the contrary, you always have to state your opinion, that is, what you believe to be right, but in a manner that does not hurt your child, does not diminish them or her, or underestimate him. Just talk.

Always show your child enough patience and time to talk. If your toddler grows up with the conviction that they still have contacts with their parents - they will feel safer and happier. Try setting priorities. If your toddler wants to talk to you while you're doing some housework, let your child do so.

Communication is learned. Occasional quarrels, conflicts, and misunderstandings are ordinary and typical occurrences in communication. But never give up.

Speech is given to us, but the conversation is learned. We all can hear, but to understand, we must put effort, time, and love into learning to listen.

How to Control the Child's Aggression

From time to time, your child gets bruises and scratches not only from taking a fall but also from playing games with their friends. Children have always played "mother and daughter" and "catch." It might seem like you could just say to your child: "Give the doll to Katie; you're a good girl!" But even if your child does it, you may not know what feelings are at work inside her: maybe they get the impression that it's not so good to be nice.

If you see or suspect how difficult it is for a two-year-old child to part with their favorite toy for the sake of good manners, it's better not to push the child and not to bring on hysterics.

When your toddler becomes a little older and has more experience in communicating, it will be easier for them or their them to focus in similar situations, and as far as possible – to try to predict them.

Often, parents are afraid of another type of situation, in which their child might be aggressive, taking a toy from another child. Almost all kids struggle if they are somewhat dissatisfied and misbehave if they are tired. Sometimes the aggressiveness of the child takes the form of your toddler biting other children. This is the same situation.

Provided a quarrel doesn't lead to outright aggression on the part of one or more of the children, parents should not interfere. If there is a need to intervene, don't try to find the culprit: for one of the children, your decision will still be unfair.

It's better to separate the fighters and divert their attention to other activities. If you see that one of the children is continually antagonizing your child, look for another circle of friends, at least for some time, where the relationship between children will be somewhat different. The same can be done if your child is too aggressive with other children.

If you observe a situation in which your two-year-old child is beating other children, don't spank them or physically discipline them in any way, and, of course, don't ask another child to do it.

Perhaps your toddler is too small to respect other children. This respect needs to be learned gradually. Take the child aside and, at the same time, explain that the other child is hurt and that your child needs to apologize to them or her. If there is an opportunity, let your bully play with older children-in that type of environment, it will be harder for them to try to prove their strength. Note: the older the child, the more selective your toddler will be regarding demonstrations of their aggressiveness towards other people. Most likely, children are aware of when they can get away with it and when they cannot.

In any case, children should be taught systematically to share toys.

If your child reveals an aggressiveness that frightens you, you should think perhaps, its origins lie in the relationships that have developed in your family. Don't forget that you are an example to your child. And yet, the skills of exhibiting a good attitude towards each other are better instilled when the child is in good humor.

Outpouring of Feelings

There is no doubt that you have an endless supply of love for your toddler.

Teach your toddler to care for everyone around them. Let them help you during cooking: put the dishes on the table with you, put out bread and fruit. And you should accompany their actions with encouraging words. Of course, it would take less time to do the work if the child wasn't "disturbing you" but you have learned that allowing them this proximity is one of your obligations as a parent. Remember this.

You might put a doll or a toy animal down to sleep, gently stroking them "before bed," saying that they've been kind and obedient. Ask your toddler to show how they or they love the doll or toy animal.

Show your toddler how to take care of flowers, paying attention to the fact that they have beautiful small and delicate leaves and flowers.

When you go for a walk, take food for birds or squirrels in the park, feed them together, and praise the toddler for it.

If the child is sad or over-excited, then perhaps they won't do what you ask of them (maybe they will break a leaf or throw a doll on the floor or won't want to feed the animals).

This temporary act of aggression does not indicate bad character traits at all.

A sense of parental love and tenderness allows a child to feel good and desired and gives him or her confidence in life.

What is Good and What is Bad

While a baby is small, the main prohibitions given by the parents are related to the concern for his or her safety. But always, when forbidding something and saying the word "No," do not forget to explain why and to tell the child how to do what they need to do. Besides, parents should know that praise is much more instructive than prohibiting things.

As often as possible, show approval for the good things your toddler does, especially those that were hard for them. Do not simply give them prohibitions. According to psychologists, verbal prohibition isn't meant for a child up to five years old.

The best solution to any problem is its joint discussion. If possible, examine the forbidden object that interests the baby together. Remembering the age of the child, try to find an explanation to show them what the danger is.

If you need to take something away from your toddler and don't let them use it, offer something to replace it, but always with something new or interesting, this way, in most cases, the conflict can be avoided.

It is advisable for adults involved in the upbringing of a child to discuss the limits allowed so that, as the toddler grows, they won't be confused when they think 'if dad considers this acceptable, why does grandma forbid it?'

But don't do this so often in the presence of the toddler. And even when being guided by safety considerations, don't forbid several things to the child at a time. This can destroy the child's desire for initiative or cause them excessive nervousness.

A child's desire to touch something with their hands or to taste it isn't always due to mischief (as sometimes it seems to parents). This is the normal desire that a child must know the world around them and to gain their own experience of things.

If you treat a child with respect, you can find many ways to manage his or her behavior. But, although you cannot do without verbal correction, you should not criticize their personality. Instead, focus on the act itself.

Try not to say to a child: **"You are bad!"** Instead, say: **"You did a bad thing!"** Even if your toddler does not understand everything, your attitude towards them and your tone of voice can make clear the meaning of what is happening.

Analyze the reasons for the conflicts that arise: is it possible that you're annoyed by seeing in your child a character trait that you have been trying to get rid of yourself for a long time?

When children are happy with everything, they usually behave well, but sometimes they unconsciously want to push the limits. Currently, it seems to parents that the child is testing their patience.

Often, bad behavior is a way to attract attention. The child may try to establish themselves as being in opposition to the adults with whom they constantly communicate. If you see the child is very enthusiastic in an activity, try not to interrupt it, even if it's time to eat or sleep.

Help them finish their "business," and then offer whatever is needed. The child will get used to finish what they are doing.

The most sensible way to resist hysterics and fits, if they become habitual, is to ignore them. Stay calm and kind with your child, but firmly insist on your authority, and in the end, your toddler will understand that lying on the floor in hysterics isn't the best way to win an argument.

It isn't necessary to send a child to another room, especially if you aren't sure about their safety. Go about your affairs, discuss other problems with your loved ones, and let the toddler remain in your field of vision. If, after some time, the child is ready for dialogue, don't reproach them for what took place a few minutes ago.

Sometimes a child needs some help to stop the hysteria.

Each family has its ways of settling disobedience, based on their experience of communicating with the child.

Try to be guided by these principles:

A child is a full member of the family (but not the center of it).

The child has the right to their own opinion (even if your toddler does not speak yet) - and this should be considered.

Just like an adult, the child has the right to a bad mood: from time to time, they may be angry, dissatisfied, or may cry. It isn't always because of external circumstances.

Chapter 10: Rules and Rewards

Establishing Rules for Your Toddler

For toddlers it's a little different because they can't conceive the concept until they are a little older, but we still work with a reward system even with the toddler. We have set rules like putting away toys before leaving a room or eating the food you don't like first. It's not easy to bring these rules into the house without a reward system in place.

Here is a list of rules and rewards we have set up for our own toddler that work:

Do not climb on the furniture

Once they can walk and talk, it's hard to get them to sit quietly and still. The talking I can still handle but the constant climbing. I am a nervous wreck. Not only because it is no place for a toddler to sit on a coffee table, but it's also very dangerous. Tables have sharp corners, chairs are high, and television cabinets contain things more expensive than the toddler's entire room. You don't want them to knock your television off the stand and you sure don't want them to knock the crystal vase from the coffee table. This is an essential rule that must be met with strict consequences.

Don't open drawers

It was wrong to despise the child so much because their them mother should have taught their them better and whenever my mother mentioned something she'd reply with "children will be children." No, ma'am. Children will most definitely not go through a stranger's personal possessions just because their parents are too lazy to teach them any better. Hence, it is a cardinal principle in my house.

Don't touch anything that doesn't belong to you

Toddlers break things. It's just the way it is. When there's a toddler in the house, it's best just to put away all the nice things and wait until they are older to take them out again. But when you visit someone else, you don't want your child's sticky hands on everything, not to mention the apologies you need to make when your child breaks something. Don't touch anything that isn't yours unless you have permission.

Don't leave a room without putting your toys away

Toddlers are messy and this carries on through their entire childhood. You must teach them from a very young age that they need to put everything away before they leave a room to keep everything neat and tidy.

No fighting

In a house with three children and one toddler, it can sometimes get a little heated. No person is the same and when there is even the smallest of disagreements, the entire house explodes into chaos. One kid hits the other with a ball of socks, the other one slams their door shut, the toddler bites and screams at whoever gets in their way. It's like a movie but without the humor.

As parents, we get exasperated. This is when each of them must go downstairs and sit at the bickering table so they can fight to their heart's content. They also get no dessert for a few days. Why? Because they know that there are better ways to settle their differences than to fight. With the tot, it can be a little rough because they can't speak their minds yet, so we just put their them in a time out after listening to their side of the story (which is usually just a load of babble and incoherent accusations), but it's crucial to let the toddler know that they are being listened to as well.

Rewarding Good Behavior

It's hard to come up with suitable rewards for your toddler. Some people go overboard with sweets and toys because they can't think about other rewards, they can give their kids. Here is an effective list of rewards that I have tried, tested, and improved to fit my tots and my pocket.

Here are some rewards I like to give my kids:

Movie of their choice

Who doesn't love a good movie on repeat? The answer is only a tot, but that's okay because at least they ate all their peas instead of tossing them at their brothers. You don't have to sit with the tot the entire time either, they get caught up in the movie and don't notice when you slip away to finish some chores in the kitchen. In general, when a tot wants to watch a movie that they have seen a hundred times, you'll tell them no, but if you give it to them as a reward, you can't refuse to let them watch it.

A trip to the zoo/museum/park

Consider your budget when you're giving out this reward. I encourage children to be outside and to explore so a park is always a good idea. They might even make some new friends while they are there! A zoo and a museum allow your tots to learn new things and words while feeling like they are getting a reward.

An extra story before bed

Bedtime stories are sometimes too short, and your tot will be asking for "just one more" on more than one occasion. Toddlers love stories and when you do not usually cave and tell them another story, this is a good way to reward them.

A game

Whether it's a toddler's board game, a puzzle, or a video game, this will be a great reward for any tot. My partner and I are both big gamers and the tot want to play along whenever we get our headsets out. Needless to say, whatever we are playing isn't suitable for a toddler.

Here is where a game on the tablet comes in. They will feel like they are joining in on the fun while not influencing your high score in the slightest. It's both a reward and a way to keep them busy while you're getting some you-time.

A cookie

The simplest thing to do is to give your child a cookie as a reward but as much as they love that, their weight and health do not. Be careful what sort of treats you give your tot and make sure that these are healthy. I usually add fruit into the cookies because my tot absolutely detests the texture of the fruit.

Chapter 11: Things to Consider When Disciplining Toddlers

Many parents attest to the reality that disciplining a toddler is like facing constant uphill battles. These little bundles of delight can turn to extremely stubborn kids who test the patience limits of caregivers and adults around them.

It is also the phase of childhood where they begin to assert their independence. One of their first words is "No," affirming the toddlers' love to do things in their way. They enjoy running away to escape. Normally, toddlers are full of energy. They run, jump, play, explore, and discover everything that interests them. They love to use the sense of touch, exploring things with their senses. Because toddlers are easily stimulated by what they see or hear, their impulsive nature can make them clumsy and touch things. Parents need to teach their children safe ways to touch or handle things and not to touch hot objects.

Although raising a toddler entails a lot of hard work, seeing your child grows and develops their skills is fascinating. However, because of the developmental changes that rapidly happen during the toddler stage, it's necessary to use a disciplinary approach that will foster the child's independence while teaching them socially appropriate behavior and other positive traits.

All too often, there is an assumption that parenting techniques apply to all, and kids will react or respond in a similar pattern. But every child has their own set of traits. This is in their DNA, which they inherited from their parents. Some toddlers are shy or even-tempered, while others are outgoing and have aggressive natures.

By understanding the child's special personality and natural behavior, you can help them adjust to the real world. It's necessary to work with their personality and not against it, considering the following factors that you need to consider when disciplining your toddler. Giving proper care and nourishment, providing positive and healthy activities, and instilling positive discipline is vital to their physical, mental, emotional, social, and behavioral growth.

Temperament and Behavior

Temperament is defined as the heritable and biologically based core that influences the style of approach and response of a person. The child's early temperament traits usually predict their adult temperament.

The child's behavior is the outcome of their temperament and the progress of their emotional, cognitive, and physical development. It is influenced by their beliefs about themself, about you, and the world in general. While it is inborn and inherent, there are certain ways to help your toddler manage it to their advantage.

Nine dimensions or traits related to temperament:

The activity level pertains to the amount of physical motion that your toddler demonstrates, while engaged in some activities. It also includes their inactive periods.

- Is your child a restless spirit that cannot sit still for long and always wants to move around?
- Is your toddler the quiet, the little one enjoys playing alone or watching TV?

Rhythmicity refers to the predictability or unpredictability of physical and biological functions which include hunger, bowel movement, and sleeping.

- Does your child thrive on routine and follow regular eating or sleeping patterns?
- DO they display unpredictable behavior and dislike routine?

Attention span and persistence are the skills to remain focused on the activity for a certain period.

- Does your toddler stick to complete a task?
- Are they easily frustrated and look for another activity?

Initial Response (Approach or Withdrawal) refers to the reaction to something new and unfamiliar. It describes their initial feelings to a stimulus like a new person, place, toy, and food. their reaction is shown by their mood or facial expressions like smiling or motor activity, such as reaching for a toy or swallowing food. Negative responses include withdrawal, crying, fussing, pushing away, or spitting the food.

- Are they wary or reluctant around unfamiliar situations or strangers?
- Do they welcome new faces and adjust comfortably

with new settings?

The intensity of reaction is associated with the level of response to any event or situation. Toddlers respond differently to events around them. Some shriek with happiness or giggle joyfully, others throw fits, and many barely react to what is happening.

- Do you always experience trying to guess the reaction of your child over something?
- Does your child explicitly show their emotions?

Adaptability is the child's ability to adjust themself to change over time.

- Is your child capable of adjusting themself to sudden changes in plans or disruptions of their routine?
- Do they find it difficult to cope up with changes and resist it as much as they can?

Distractibility is the level of the child's willingness to be distracted. It relates to the effects of an outside stimulus on your child's behavior.

- Can your child focus on their activity despite the distraction that surrounds him?
- Are they unable to concentrate when there are people or other activities going on in the environment?

Quality of mood is related to how your child sees the world in their own eyes and understanding. Some react with acceptance and pleasure while other children scowl with displeasure just "because" they feel like it.

- Do they display mood changes constantly?
- Do they generally have a happy disposition?

Sensory Threshold is linked to sensitivity to sensory stimulation. Children who are sensitive to stimulation requires a careful and gradual introduction to new people, experiences, or objects.

- Is your child easily bothered by bright lights, loud sounds, or food textures?
- Are they totally undisturbed with such things and welcome them as such?

There are three main types of toddlers:

- Active or Feisty Toddlers- These children have a tremendous amount of energy, which they show even while inside the uterus of their mothers, like lots of moving and kicking. As an infant, they move around, squirm, and crawl all over the place. As toddlers, they climb, run, jump, and even fidget a lot to release their energy. They become excited while doing things or anxious around strangers or new situations.

They are naturally energetic, joyful, and loves fun. But when they are not happy, they will clearly and loudly say it. These toddlers are also quite obstinate and hard to fit in regular routines.

To help them succeed:

- Acknowledge their unique temperament and understand their triggers.
- Teach them self-help skills to get going if their energy is low or how to calm down when their activity level is very high. Some simple and effective ways to calm down are counting from 1 to 10, taking deep breaths, doing jumping jacks to get rid of excess energy, and redirecting them to other activities.
- Set a daily routine that includes play and other activities that enhance their gross motor movements. Provide them with opportunities to play and explore safely. It is necessary to childproof your home.
- Insist on nap time. An afternoon nap will refresh their body and mind, preventing mood swings and tantrums.
- Do not let them sit in front of a television or do

passive activities. Break the boredom by taking them outside and play in the outdoors.

➤ Become a calming influence. Understand how your temperament affects their temperament and find ways to become a role model.

• Passive or Cautious Toddlers- These children prefer activities that don't require a lot of physical effort, move slower, and want to sit down more often. They are slow-to-warm-up when meeting new people and often withdraw when faced with an unfamiliar situation. They also need ample time to complete their tasks.

To help them succeed:

➤ If your child is less active, set guidelines or deadlines that will prompt them to finish the given tasks.

➤ Invite them to play actively by using interesting sounds, bright toys, or gentle persuasion.

➤ Always accentuate the positive. Be generous with praise and words of encouragement when they display efforts or achieve simple milestones.

• Flexible or Easy Toddlers - These children are very adaptable, generally calm, and happy. But sometimes, they are easily distracted and need a lot of reassurance and love from you.

To help them succeed:

➤ Be realistic and expect mood changes when something isn't smooth sailing. Don't be too hard on the child when they display unusual outburst.

➤ Provide them with interactive activities and join him. Sometimes, it's easy to let them play their own devices because of their good-natured personality. It is necessary to introduce other options to enhance their skills.

➤ Read the signs and find out the reasons for subtle changes in the behavior and attitude toward something. Be observant and have a special time for him.

B. Nine Methods for Toddler Discipline

Instilling discipline is a dilemma for most parents, especially the new ones. They look for the most effective approach to raise well-mannered and positive children who can cope up with the challenges in the real world.

Technically, there is no right or wrong approach except the punitive ways that scar children for life. All it takes is to find the right disciplinary method that will work with your child's inherent personality, behavior, and temperament.

Chapter 12: Manners and Following Directions

Remember those days when the boys were sent off to boarding schools? They always looked so groomed when they returned, didn't they? So knowledgeable and polished. There were many such schools in Boston and London, aimed at transforming adolescents into gracious adults. They had to abide by many strict rules, give up damaging habits and develop ones that helped them build their personality and character. Maybe you married one such adult or are one yourself. Nonetheless, now that you're a parent and see your nine-year-old depicting behaviors that were considered a cardinal sin back then, you must wonder where did you fall short? Why did your child grow up this cranky, and ill-mannered?

And forget about boarding schools, we seemed to have it all under control during our childhood. Of course, we were naughty, but our level of naughty was way less. We were well-mannered, had basic etiquettes and rarely did anything to upset or embarrass our parents. Because god forbid, they notice and give us the stare!

Since kids aren't born with the innate ability to learn a language, imitate behaviors and repeat actions, it has to be on us. We must have done something or not done something to raise them the way they are. If they aren't polite, it is be on us. If they aren't disciplined and obedient, it has to be our fault, right? Yes and no.

Learning to Behave and Becoming Well-Mannered

The ability to act decent, with grace and politely is another great social skill to have. Good manners refer to the set of behaviors and actions that someone exhibits out of habit. For example, saying sorry when they hit someone, starting the question with "please" when requesting something or replying with a "thank you" when their request is fulfilled.

Why is Good Manners and Discipline Important?

There is more than just one reason to teach your children good manners and lead their life with discipline. For starters, good manners should be a way of life. We shouldn't just teach our kids to behave well at social gatherings but teach them to act civil and responsible at all times. The best way is to begin early as a habit picked up early on is hard to let go if they are bad ones. Therefore, if they have been exposed to bad manners and a lack of discipline in the house, chances are they are going to pick up the same. This will lead them to trouble in places like schools, public events, and even weddings and restaurants. Not to mention, you'll be the one to have to deal with the display of bad manners. Other than that: Good manners or social graces help develop other social skills. Remember the time when your child was in kindergarten? Did you ever send them to school without a healthy snack or lunch? Social graces are the same. When kids who lack basic manners, go out in the world, they become a major turn-off to others, especially the kids their age. They may not mind your child taking their toy without permission, but they will start to when your child refuses to give it back or respond with hitting or biting. This example shows that your child lacks manners, and everyone will be quick to point it out.

Activities to Instill Good Manners at an Early Age

By now, you must be desperately looking forward to this section, as we may have scared you a little bit. Well, worry not, these games and activities are the perfect way to teach them about something so vital and yet don't make them realize that they are being schooled.

Question Time To encourage good behavior and manners, you must first know how much work you need to do and where you need to begin with. Think of this not as a game, but rather a reality check for you as a parent. In this first exercise, you're going to ask them a series of questions to check for their responses. You start by offering them made-up scenarios and ask them to respond with "how will they deal with it." For example, how will they deal/respond:

• When someone walks in front of you?

o Ask them politely to excuse you, or o Push them and move forward

• When someone sits too close to them?

o Push them aside, or o Make room for them by moving to the other side

- When someone wants the toy you are playing with?
- ○ Give it to them, or ○ Refuse to share or take turns
- When someone gives you something?
- ○ Say thank you, or ○ Take it without saying thank you.

DIY Manners Box In this activity, start with cutting a few colored printer sheets into small three-inch coins or squares. Write one good manner on each sheet of paper and place it beside an empty jar with an open slid in the lid to push the sheets inside. Tell your child to put one sheet in the jar whenever they perform the good action written on it. The examples you can write on the little sheets can be the following:

- I said, thank you
- I said sorry
- I said please
- I shared my toy with my sibling
- I changed into my night clothes myself
- I watched 1 hour of TV today
- I completed all my homework
- I knocked on the door before entering the room
- I greeted everyone when entering the house
- I covered my mouth when I sneezed/coughed
- I washed my hands before every meal
- I brushed my teeth before going to bed etc.

Set a reward if they add 5+ sheets of paper in the jar by the end of the day. You'll notice how eager they will be to perform these actions. Soon, all these activities will turn into a life-long habit.

Manners Tea Party-To teach basic eating and dining out manners, invite them to a tea party to portray basic dining etiquettes. Show them how awful it looks when they run around a restaurant, smash plates, make noise and disturb others. Show them how the whole scene can be as calm and elegant.

Practice Phone Manners Phone manners, like table or communication manners, are also important. They teach kids how to respond on the phone politely. Pretend to have a call with them, several times during the day and teach them what to say by offering them different situations. For example, you can call in to say that you are a friend of theirs and that you need to borrow their school copy as they are facing trouble with the homework. Or you can act like you're a relative that wants to talk to your mother or father. Teach them the basics first and then show them how they can improvise.

Tell them to always greet the person with a gracious greeting like, 'hello' or 'hi.' Then, ask them their name and purpose of the call like, "May I know who is calling?" or "Who do you want to speak to?" and then tell the caller to wait until you get your father/mother to the phone.

Rate Them If you want to instill good behavior and manners in your child, you must know what intrigues them. Praises, compliments, and acknowledgment are some of the most rewarding ways to get them to do something. It is no secret that every child wishes to impress their parents. It's like a goal they need to achieve. Thus, they resort to behaviors and actions they notice you like or praise.

This activity, however, takes it up a notch. Here you not only praise them for their effort but also let others know about it. All you need is a sheet of paper with their name on it and a few stickers in the shape of a heart or stars. You make a list of chores you want them to do or behaviors you want them to demonstrate and once they do them, you give them a star right beside the chore or behavior. The more stars they get, the bigger the reward. The rewards don't have to be something tangible always. It can also be things like 15-minutes extra of TV watching or getting their favorite dessert after dinner etc.

Additional Tips and Info

Whether you believe it or not, a well-mannered child stands out for their discipline and politeness. Teaching good manners isn't hard and just a little practice and repetition of good manners does the job. Here are a few tips to get you started!

• Encourage the use of words like "please," "thank you," and "sorry."

• Set rewards for your children when they respond with politeness and exhibit good table, communication, or playing manners.

- Don't forget to boost their ego and foster repetition of certain good behavior by complimenting and praising it. They will likely do it again, just to impress you.
- When taking them someplace, let them know what is expected of them before you leave the house. Also, subtly highlight any repercussions for bad behavior such as not getting an ice-cream on the way back home if they misbehave.
- But when listing your expectations, make them age appropriate. You can't expect them to stay seated when every other kid is having the time of their lives in the jumping castle.

Chapter 13: Methods for Toddler Discipline

Instilling discipline is a dilemma for most parents, especially the new ones. They look for the most effective approach to raise well-mannered and positive children capable of coping with the challenges in the real world.

Technically, there is no right or wrong approach except the punitive ways that scar children for life. All it takes is to find the right disciplinary 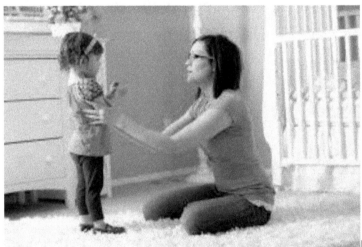method that will work with your child's inherent personality, behavior, and temperament.

Here are some simple methods that are widely used by parents all over the world:

Commendation & Encouragement

Praise and encouraging words always bring positive outcomes, motivating toddlers to show good behavior. Giving your child small rewards or applause when they do something commendable will encourage them to continue improving their skills. Praising good behaviors will make them repeat the same thing to gain your approval and praise.

Rethinking

Changing the tone of your discourse or reframing your thoughts often results in a positive reaction. Instead of giving an instruction that uses "don't do that" or "gets that" rethink your strategy to mirror solicitation. It's better to use the phrases, "would you...if it is fine with you?"

Remember that your toddler is not a mini-you. It also helps to view things from their perspective. For instance, they do not want to sit in the child's car seat. You may say- "I know that you do really like sitting in your car seat, but it's essentially like this seat belt that I have. They make us both safe." In this manner, you are teaching them the importance of being safe by using proper tools.

Disregard

Disregarding fits or tantrums intentionally sends a clear signal to your child that you are not affected by their behavior, and you will not succumb to their whims. To make it more effective, all other adults in your home must know this strategy to discipline and break the child's tantrum habits. It may seem harsh but refraining to engage or respond to your child's temper tantrum is one of the keys to curb the practice.

Ignoring or looking the other way is an effective way to curb the child's habit of doing something naughty just to get your attention. Avoid meeting their eyes, glaring, or getting angry because it signifies that your attention to him. You need to act like you are not disturbed by their behavior, making them realize that screaming or throwing tantrums will not make you yield to their desires.

Break

It is also called a timeout, a popular technique most parents used to discipline their children. The idea is to send them to a specific "cozy spot" in your home, a place that is safe and free from stimulation or distraction and let them reflect on their behavior. It's essential that you can see them and ensure their safety. After a specific time of the break, talk about what happened, giving them time to explain and admit their misdeed.

A good rule of thumb for setting a time limit must correspond to the child's age, so if your kid is two years old, enforce a 2-minute break. But try to use this method sparingly and avoid making them feel isolated or alone.

Substitute & Distraction

If your child has this habit of hitting something inside the house like banging their toy on the table, distract them before they can do it. You can attract their attention by showing them something. Young children are easy to distract because they usually have a short attention span. You can also substitute their toys, redirecting them into something more interesting.

Toddlers don't understand why they have to be disciplined. Divert their attention with another activity or toy that will interest him. Calling their name aloud for their attention, then once their eyes fixate on you, show them something that will compel them to come to you.

Offer Decisions

Letting your child take part in simple decision-making like the color of the shirt they want to wear gives them a sense of pride and control. It boosts their confidence and lessens the occurrences of power struggles. By involving them in the process, you ease the transition and make them proud of making a choice.

These last three methods should avoid as much as possible.

Surrendering to fits of rage

Your little child will be persistent and throw fits of anger to make you give in to their demands. If you yield the first time, it becomes a ticket for them to attempt another try. It is the toddler's control strategy and can be prevented by not generating to their unreasonable requests that will compromise their health and safety.

Raising your voice. When is it appropriate?

Some parents admit that sometimes, they yell at their children. Studies show that yelling is one of the discipline techniques that can make behavior issues worse, undermining the parent and child bond. It also loses its effectiveness over time when your child begins to tune you out when you do it regularly.

When is yelling necessary? Expressing your emotions aloud can be positive for you and your child, helping them develop empathy and realize that they have upset you. Although, be mindful of your language. Instead of "you" statements, use "I" statements like "I am feeling disappointed because you won't share your toys with your brother" rather than "You are not nice!" It is also necessary to be aware of your feelings and behavior. Sometimes, you bellow out because you're in a bad mood or tired, and not because your child has done something wrong.

Punishment

Punishment in all forms, including spanking, caning, and beating, is a big NO. It has been a thing in the past that parents used to control their children, but many studies showed that it caused long-term disdain and misery. Spanking, for example, even occasional, can lead to the development of childhood anxiety and makes your child think that it's fine to hit.

Children learn to be afraid of the consequences when caught but do it anyway when you are not present. If you say, "Don't make me catch you doing it again or you will ground!" they may interpret the act as not inappropriate, and they just needs to be careful so you'll catch them doing it. The result does not resolve the behavior problem and becomes ineffective in helping the child make better choices or learn self-control. There is also a consistent result in various surveys that punishment pushes children to spend more time avoiding behavior and being rebellious.

Chapter 14: Effective Techniques That Can Turn Any Negative Behavior into A Positive One

Effective discipline is composed of a system of techniques or strategies that aim to suppress bad behavior and teach the right conduct. There are many techniques that you can try. But, with so many techniques to choose from, how do you know which one works? Through years of trial and error, the following techniques have proven effective in disciplining toddlers.

Distract

When your toddler does something unacceptable, you can call their attention to something else. For example, if they keep on nagging and screaming, you can offer them a toy or read their favorite book with him. If they get annoying while playing a game, you can switch to a different game or maybe put the TV on their favorite channel. Usually, toddlers are well behaved when they are satisfied and happy.

Say No

As a parent, it feels right and normal to give everything that your toddler asks for. Therefore, as much as you can, you're always inclined to say yes. Though, you need to understand the importance of saying no. Sometimes, the word no is as significant, if not more, than saying yes. It is not that you cannot give your child what they want, but always spoiling your child with a 'yes' can be a major problem. Your child must learn at an early age that they cannot always have everything that they want instantly. Of course, you should not deprive your child of good and healthy things. But, for example, if you're at a mall and they ask for candy, you should also learn to say no from time to time.

The problem is that many parents tend to spoil their child with yeses then complain when their child lashes out at them. Just as you must discipline your child, you should also discipline yourself. Teach your child how to handle little frustrations by saying no.

This technique isn't only limited to saying no. You can also say stop if your toddler does something that you do not like. Also, something that is very useful to learn is to ignore your toddler. Ignoring your toddler is recommended, especially when they do silly, undesirable things just to catch attention.

You should, however, avoid saying no many times, especially in succession. Even an adult who receives a negative response many times would feel frustrated. To lighten things up, what you can do is to use an alternative. You can do this by offering a substitute. For example, if you need your kid to take a break from watching TV, you can offer a book or a toy for their enjoyment. You must understand that kids always need to be doing something; otherwise, they will get bored and start misbehaving.

Saying no also helps when you want a certain behavior to be suppressed, for example, "no biting" or "no running." The trick here is for you not to make a big deal out of it. Just say it clearly and then switch to another topic or focus. The key is to bring the message across to your child without making a big deal out of it.

Positive reinforcement

Traits or behaviors that are ignored or suppressed tend to fade away and disappear, while those that are rewarded get reinforced and remain. Reinforcement is of two kinds: negative and positive. Negative reinforcement is when you give a mild punishment for every undesirable behavior, while positive reinforcement is when you reward good behaviors. It's best to focus on positive reinforcement than negative reinforcement. Take note that discipline isn't just about removing or suppressing a behavior; more significantly, it also means teaching the right behavior.

The rewards do not have to be expensive. They don't always have to be in material form. Giving praise or expressing appreciation — such as "Thank you. You are so kind." or "I am proud of you." — works well too and matters a lot. Be sure to be sincere about it. Mean what you say.

According to a study, positive reinforcement is better than discipline by punishment. The study shows that, on the one hand, more parts of the brain are needed to function for a toddler to understand the true purpose of punishment fully. More analysis would be needed, which isn't a recommended method in dealing with an adult. On the other hand, positive reinforcement is very easy for toddlers to connect to, and it's effective in strengthening the behavior that is being enforced. Even their minds easily understand how positive reinforcement works without a problem.

Defensive parenting

Parents don't need to exercise any discipline when there is no reason to do so. This technique relies on prevention than a cure. By removing the things and avoiding the occasions that tend to make your child misbehave, there will be fewer problems for you. Sometimes toddlers can try your patience. If you think you already have many issues with your child, then using defensive parenting can lighten things up. This also includes not talking to your child in a way that will annoy him. If you think a certain word or sound irritates him, then avoid using it.

To apply this properly, you need to be attentive to the things that annoy your child or make them act inappropriately, so you'll know the things that should be avoided. Defensive parenting requires that you take notice and respond accordingly. Pay attention to what triggers your child's inappropriate behavior and take the time to understand why it happens. Is there anything you can do so that it can be avoided? If you cannot completely remove what triggers the wrong behavior, find a way to decrease the effect of such stimuli somehow.

Logical consequences

Toddlers don't usually care about the consequences of their actions. This technique will teach your toddler how to understand the outcome of their actions and take responsibility. This can be as simple as making them brush their teeth after eating or cleaning their mess when they spill their milk. By doing so, they get to understand the consequences of their actions and also become more responsible. Of course, this should be controlled. If the mess is too much for your child to clean all by themself, then help out. This technique isn't a license to getting your kid always to fix their mess. This technique aims to make your kid understand the consequences of their actions, and not merely as a way of punishment.

Correct the behavior, not the child

Always remember that your job is to change the behavior. Whether your toddler keeps screaming or displays other negative behaviors, you should deal with the behavior. It helps to understand and separate the negative behavior from the child. Having such an understanding will also help you control your temper.

It is also worth noting that toddlers are very sensitive. They don't like being blamed or pressured. So, instead of saying, "You are a bad kid." whenever they scream or misbehaves, say, "Stop. Screaming is wrong." or whatever the action is.

By separating the inappropriate behavior from the child, you can more effectively deal with the problem. Even your child would see it as something that isn't part of who they is, and so, they or they can more easily exercise control over the wrong behavior.

Be a good example

Children look up to their parents even when they don't say anything about it. They observe your actions, your words, gestures, and how you interact with people. If there is anything in the world that has the strongest influence on them, then it would be you. So, be a good example. Your toddler would not know what kindness is unless you show it to him. In the same way, teach your child the beauty of forgiveness by being forgiving yourself.

This isn't a one-time thing. Being a good example means living it, being respectful, and upright with your ways. Since your kid will always take notice of you, you cannot expect to discipline your kids to be loving and respectful if you don't observe such values. By simply being a good example, you help shape your toddler into a good adult that they will be. Take note that this technique does not only refer to your relationship with your toddler. Your kid also notices how you interact with other people; so, be sure to treat your spouse, family members, and friends nicely.

It isn't easy to be a good example, especially when you encounter some bad days at work or simply a string of bad luck in life. Although, you should maintain your composure and stay calm, at least do so when your child can see you. If the pressure is too much for you to handle, you might as well hide from your toddler. The important thing is that you should always appear good, kind, and pleasant before your child's eyes. Keep in mind that whatever toddlers see, especially what they see from their parents, have a big impact on their behavior. This is another reason why it is not good to quarrel with your spouse in front of your kids. Remember: No matter how silly they may appear; toddlers are very sensitive. Be sure to pay attention to the things that they see, hear, and feel.

It should be noted that changing behavior, specifically from negative into positive, takes time. Do not be hard on your child and yourself if the behavior repeats a few more times. It usually takes weeks before a person can completely change a certain behavior, especially when such behavior has already become a habit. But don't lose hope because change is always possible. Even at your age, change is very much possible.

Chapter 15: How to Praise Effectively

As your kid grows and starts to grasp the connection amid their actions and outcomes, be sure you begin praising and compensating your children on behalf of their achievements. The main purpose of doing so is towards increasing the motivation of your children.

Once praising children, it's significant to put emphasis on their hard work and achievements. Before doing this, explain to your kid whatever you require of them prior to any punishment or reward. Consistency exists as the secret to effective punishment and reward system.

So, it's vital that parents decide what the home rules are, as well as upholding them. When everything is clear to the children, then the use of encouraging words for kids become effective. After all, discipline isn't just about chastisement, but also on recognizing good conduct.

In the example in the preceding chapter, I never failed to tell my child how proud I am of them for tidying up their toys after playing. In this way, I make it obvious which behaviors I like and why. This causes such conduct to be more expected to occur in the days to come, and the more awareness parents provide to a conduct, the more prone it stays to continue.

You know you are praising your child effectively when you're:

Avoiding calculating, comparison or conditional admiration.

When praise stays used by way of a controlling means, they utter support and positive assessment, which is dependent on good performance. These provisional encouragements impart a feeling of contingent self-esteem in kids.

This is illustrated when a child feels that their self-respect is influenced by how good they play volleyball. As a result, their goals would be to do well in training and matches towards increasing or maintaining a positive self-confidence. Also, she'll avoid any activity that may end in negative assessment.

Commending your child's hard work and the course of action, not the child's ability.

This means praising your kid for knowing how to control naughtiness and particularly for overcoming a stubborn problem. Instead of saying, "The best painter," say, "My, you must have spent countless hours honing your painting skills!"

Praising honestly.

At all times, praise should be genuine. Children have a technique of perceiving when your approval is insincere. When they sense you're insincere, you'll lose their trust and they may become insecure. When they doubt your positive comments, they will find it difficult to tell the difference amid when you truly mean what you're saying and at what time you do not.

Specific and imaginative in your praises.

Instead of "You are such a great volleyball player," say, "You can really smash the ball hard to make it difficult for the other team to handle it!" Being specific exists much better, besides helping kids identify their special talent.

Steering clear of overly praising your child.

Praising easy chores imply that you really don't expect much from your child. Although praises given unexpectedly can be extremely motivating, overpraising, on the other hand, conditions children anticipate some words of encouragement each time. It converts an extrinsic gift into something that reduces motivation.

Frequent complementing also leads kids to believe that its absence signifies failure. Just as huge punishments can remove your authority as a father or a mother, it equally has the opposite effect when you praise your child.

Chapter 16: Common Mistakes That Parents Make and How to Fix Them

Disciplining your toddlers alone is not alone. You must also avoid the common pitfalls of parenting. Many of these blunders don't just decrease the effectiveness of the discipline that you impose on your toddler but may even encourage your toddlers to misbehave. Here are the common mistakes that many parents make when disciplining their children.

Being Aggressive

Some parents simply give up and become aggressive. The problem with being aggressive is that the children learn nothing except fear. They don't get to understand the value that you want them to learn. Instead, they obey you out of fear. Studies also show that toddlers who have experienced aggressive or abusive parents are likely to grow aggressive as well. Being aggressive does not just mean spanking your kids, but it also includes using highly offensive words and threatening words. It's important to note that you are dealing with a toddler and being aggressive is the worst thing you can do.

Comparing Yourself with Other Parents

Stop comparing yourself with other parents. How they discipline their kids is their problem. If one of your friends tells you that slapping your kid in the face is effective, even if they could prove it, don't follow the advice blindly. After all, according to various studies, slapping or hitting your kids isn't an effective way to discipline them.

Comparing your Child with Other Children

It is wrong to compare your child with other children, except if it will be something that will make them feel good about themself. Would you like your child to compare you in terms of money with a parent who is much richer than you are? Of course not. In the same way, you should not compare your child with other children. Your toddler is unique in their way, and you should appreciate them as they are.

Lying

Some parents lie to their toddlers to make them obey. Although this may work from time to time, it also has bad consequences. In a case study of a mom from New Jersey with a 2-year-old daughter, it so happened that one day her child refused to get into the car, she pointed at her neighbor's house nearby and told her kid that it was a daycare center full of troglodytes from a scary TV show. She told her daughter that she had two choices, to get in the car or be left alone in the house with a threat of being attacked by creepy cavemen. Of course, her daughter finally gave in and entered the car. Now, if you look at what happened, it will seem that it was successful. There was no shouting or spanking or anything that took place. However, the problem here occurred after the incident. Following the case study, the mom's daughter began to have a fear of daycare centers, thinking that such places have scary cavemen. As you can see, even when the mother was able to make her child to do what was needed, the consequence was worse. Thus, instead of lying, the best way is, to be honest, and be emphatic.

Yelling

You don't have to yell at your toddler just to get your point across. According to Dr. Alan Greene, a pediatrician and member of the clinical faculty at Stanford University School of Medicine, if you lose control and start yelling, your kid will also do the same. Now, this does not mean that your kid is intentionally disrespecting you. This only proves that your child is having a hard time with you because you cannot understand each other. Hence, you must keep your voice quiet yet firm. Eyes contact also helps.

Thinking that You Understand Your Toddler

The truth is that you cannot always understand your toddler. This is simply because toddlers don't think the same way as adults do. You simply cannot tell exactly how certain things have an impact on your toddler's feelings and thoughts. More significantly, you do not know just up to what degree. Therefore, don't be too hard on your toddler.

Raising the Child, you Want

Do not impose your life or your will upon your toddler. Your child has their own life. Let them pursue whatever they want. Let them paint their dreams and believe in them. Focus on the child whom you already have and not the idea of a child in your mind whom you would wish to have. Your child may not be wired the way you would want them to be, and this is normal. Let your child have their chance in life. Let them believe and live their dreams.

Correcting Everything at the Same Time

Many parents try to correct all the inappropriate behaviors of their child, and they expect a toddler to be able to do it within a short period. This is a very unreasonable expectation. Even you cannot change your bad manners and behaviors quickly, so don't expect your toddler to be able to do it much more than you can. Not to mention, most parents' complaint about their toddlers with normal behaviors or misbehaviors.

You must learn to pick your battles, and don't even attempt to win everything at the same time. You may start with the behavior that you consider to be the most serious and requires attention. Once you have corrected it, then you can move to another. Of course, you should discipline your child with every opportunity that presents itself. But learn to focus on a behavior, so you can also gauge the effectiveness of the technique or techniques that you are using.

Long Explanations

Long explanations do not work on toddlers. You will only seem like talking gibberish after a few minutes. Don't forget that toddlers have a short attention span; thus, long explanations don't work well with them. For example, you don't have to lecture your toddler why eating cookies before bedtime isn't good for their them teeth. they will learn that when the right time comes. Instead, just say, "No cookies." You don't have to explain so much. After all, toddlers aren't meant to be very logical. They don't care so much about explanations. Of course, this rule is subject to exceptions, such as when the toddler themself wants to know the reason behind something or when giving an explanation appears to be the best course of action.

Bribe

Do not bribe your toddler just to make them do what you want. Otherwise, they will always ask for it, which could be a problem in the long run. In a case study of a mom in Montclair, New Jersey, she offered her daughter a piece of chocolate if she (her toddler) would eat her meal. It worked well. Her daughter finished her meal quickly. Up to this point, it would seem that bribing is also effective. Although, what happened here was that after that dinner, the daughter would always ask her mother to give her a piece of chocolate so that she would finish her meal.

Instead of bribing your child, the suggested way is to help them realize the importance of food. Using the case as mentioned earlier study, the better way would be to tell her child that she will get hungry late in the evening if she eats so little and that she will not be healthy, which could make her sick. If you face a similar problem with your child, you can tell them about the health benefits of the food, like it could make their skin more beautiful, make them taller or smarter, or stronger and powerful — but do not lie.

Not Asking Questions

Toddlers usually have so many questions. As a parent, you tend to answer your question as much as you can. It's worth noting that you should not lie to your child when they ask questions. Though, you can make silly answers, but be sure that they know that it's a joke when you do so. Also, avoid giving creepy answers or those that will tend to scare your child. So, avoid answers that relate to ghosts and other scary stuff. However, parents get too caught up with answering their child's countless questions that they miss another beneficial thing to do: to ask their child questions.

If you can take the time to ask your toddler questions, even crazy and illogical ones, you might just be surprised by the answers that you might hear. Toddlers have a powerful imagination and are very curious and open to almost everything. By asking questions to your child, you will also get to understand how they thinks, and even appreciate how young they truly is — so all the more reason why you should never be aggressive or harsh on your toddler.

Chapter 17: How to Handle Temper Tantrums

Children express their frustrations with various challenges through tantrums. Maybe your toddler is having difficulties in completing a specific task? Perhaps they don't have the right words to express what they feel? Frustrations play a major role in triggering anger that leads to tantrums. Let's look at various ways to handle tantrums in children.

Take the right steps to prevent the tantrums.

Schedule some frequent playtime with your little one. Allow them to choose the activity and make sure the child gets complete attention from you. Sharing a positive experience will offer your child an excellent foundation to calm themself down whenever they get upset. Observe the opportunities that acknowledge their excellent performance. When a child receives favorable attention for the desired performance, they'll then form a habit of doing the same.

You can also create good tactics to deal with the frustrations immediately, like taking a deep breath. It's also essential to

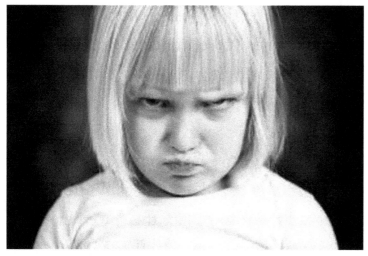

fess up after being angry over something. That's because your child needs to know it's OK to make mistakes occasionally. Make sure you know the things that lead to the tantrum and plan well. If the child gets frustrated when they're hungry, try to carry some healthy snacks. If the child starts grumbling when tired, try to make sleep time a priority.

Speak whenever the child yells

Your toddler will match the tone of your voice since they want to get your attention. Bear in mind, and they're feeling angry and sad might assist you to remain calm. Whenever they lose control at a public spot such as the movies, take the child outside. Allow them to sit on the bench or in the car as they settle down. For most children, having such choices will help, mainly if the lack of control causes the outburst.

After an episode, try to follow through with the first demand that caused it. If the child became frustrated because you asked them to collect the toy, they could still get it when they're calm. If the child started screaming because you didn't allow them to have a cookie, then give the cookie once they stop crying. When the child follows through and collects the toy, applaud the child. That's because it's a positive habit you'll want to instill in them.

Know why your toddler reacts strongly.

While your child can use words to express what they want, that doesn't imply that the tantrums have ended. They're still learning ways to handle emotions, and a slight disagreement will make them frustrated and sad. Since your toddler values their growing independence, requiring your help might be frustrating. They might break down when trying to complete a challenging task such as tying shoelaces and they realize they cannot do it by themselves. Even though tantrums tend to start with anger, they're always deep-rooted in sadness. Children might get lost in how unjust, and huge a situation becomes, so they struggle with how to do the task successfully.

Attempt this one tactic for tantrums for children below two and a half years. In most cases, children within this age bracket have 50 words in their vocabulary and can't link over two words together at a time. The child's communication is limited, but they have countless thoughts, needs, and wishes that must be met. When you fail to understand what they want, they tend to freak out to express their sadness and frustration. The remedy for this is to teach the children how to sign some words like milk, food, and tired. Empathizing with your child is another method to deal with outbursts. It assists in curbing the tantrums.

Give your child some space and create a diversion.

In most cases, a child is supposed to get rid of the anger. So, just let them do it. This method will help your child know how to vent in a non-destructive manner. They'll have a chance to release their feelings, get themselves together, and recover self-control. Your child will engage in a yelling contest or fight with you. This approach can work in tandem with ignoring it a bit.

This entails a definite mental switcheroo. Try to get your child engaged and interested in other things to make them forget about the bad experience. Make sure your backpack or purse has all kinds of distractions such as toys, comic books, and yummy snacks. Once your child starts throwing tantrums, get the distraction out to catch your child's attention.

Note that a distraction can assist you in warding off a huge outburst before it occurs, provided you catch it in time. If you sense your child is about to scream at the store after you tell them you won't buy them what they want, try to switch gears and enthusiastically say something such as "Hey, do we need some bread. Do you want to assist me in getting the things on the list?" children tend to have a short attention duration, and this makes it easy to divert their attention. When doing this, make sure you sound psyched as it will make your child know it's real. They'll tend to forget about what made them feel sad and focus on the next better thing.

Offer a big and tight hug.

This might feel the hardest thing to do when your toddler is acting up, but it'll help them calm down. This should be a big tight hug and never say anything when doing it. Hugs will make your child feel secure and allow them to understand you care about them, even though you don't support the tantrum habits. In most cases, a child needs a safe place to release one's emotions.

Give them food or suggest some R&R

Getting tired and being hungry is the leading cause of tantrums in children. Since the child is on the brink emotionally, an outburst will quickly occur. Most parents keep wondering why their child has meltdowns that occur during the same time every day—for instance, many toddler's tantrums before lunch and in the evening, which is never a coincidence. If you're experiencing this, make sure you feed your child well and give them enough water. After that, let them veg, whether it involves taking them to bed or letting them watch TV.

Give the child incentive to behave.

Some situations are trying for children. They can encompass sitting for long hours in a restaurant when eating or staying calm in church. Irrespective of the scenario, the tactic is about noticing when you're asking for too much from your child. Also, remember to give them the incentive for the good work done. While heading to the restaurant, for instance, tell her," Maya, mom wants you to sit and take your dinner nicely. I know you'll do that! And if you behave well, you'll play your video games when we get home. This type of bribery is perfectly provided. It's done as per your terms and before time and not under pressure in the middle of a tantrum. In case they begin to lose their temper, remind them about your promise. It's great how it'll suddenly guide them back into shape.

Laugh it off

As a parent, you fear public tantrums for various reasons. You're probably afraid other people will brand you a bad parent, or that you're raising an out of control child. But that might lure you into making some choice that will result in deep fits. Children are always smart, even the little ones. If you get stressed and angry, allow them to find the best way to end the outburst before many people begin staring, they'll learn on their own. The best thing is to suck it up, put on a smile, and pretend that everything is OK.

Get out of that place

Getting your little one away from the place of a tantrum will subdue the outburst. Additionally, it's an ideal strategy when you're in public places. When your child starts yelling over candy bars or a toy they want, take the child to a different place within the supermarket or even outside until they stop crying. Shifting the place will likely change the behavior.

Daily Life of your Toddler

There is no doubt about it, the toddler years are a time of immense learning, growing, and development. There are so many things that our toddlers are learning daily, and parents and caregivers are responsible for providing the structure and the tools for success as our toddlers explore their worlds and learn how to make sense of each day as it comes.

Parents and caregivers of toddlers know that each day is ripe with opportunities to guide and teach our little ones to complete their daily tasks, such as eating, playing, relating to others, and sleeping. Loving and respectful discipline includes the guidance and structure that gives toddlers the tools they need to be successful in these areas.

Eating Habits

If we were to take a poll of toddler parents and enquire into their daily eating habits, it would be expected that there would be many that would lament their toddler's appetite fluctuations or their pickiness and preferences, or perhaps their table manners. This is all too common, particularly in Western culture. There are some cultural reasons for this. In Western culture, it's common for toddlers to be served food throughout the day, in small snacking amounts, but then to also be expected to sit through the standard family meals three times a day, even when they aren't all that hungry and when they have not been expected to sit still for that length of time and eat that much in that sort of setting. It's also common for toddlers to often be given the bland, tasteless, and soft textured foods marketed towards them, rather than allowing them to explore and learn a variety of tastes and textures. There is also often a certain element of pressure and power struggle that accompanies mealtimes with toddlers that creates more struggle and negative associations around mealtimes than is necessary or helpful.

To begin, it can be helpful to reframe how we feel about our toddler's eating habits into a loving and respectful discipline mindset. These early toddler years are an excellent time for parents and caregivers to facilitate a healthy relationship between their toddlers and food. Power struggles and pressure only serve to create angst and anxiety around eating and food choices and contribute to picky and resistant future eaters as well.

A healthy relationship with food is one in which food is being used for nourishment and health, and not for comfort and appeasement of others. If we set up a dynamic in which our toddlers are being forced to eat a certain amount of food to appease us and meet an arbitrary guideline, then we are teaching them that their relationship to food is externally driven, rather than an intuitive practice in which they ingest food for their nourishment and health.

This is one of the spots that can become particularly tricky for parents and caregivers. To begin with, we all know that our toddlers must eat! How is it then, that there are days where our toddlers seem quite content to exist on a handful of cheerios and nothing more? This is completely normal. Toddler appetites can fluctuate wildly, both day-to-day and meal-to-meal. This is due in large part because their little bodies are going through growth spurts, or periods of expedited growth, that can require a boost in calorie intake, and then once the growth spurt has ended, they go back to their previous calorie requirements. There is also the daily distraction of a new and shiny world that they are desperate to explore that can also make it easy for them to prioritize playing over sitting down to eat a full meal.

There is a healthy eating model called the Division of Responsibility in Feeding that is recommended by several leading health agencies, including The Academy of Nutrition and Dietetics, The American Academy of Pediatrics, the Expert Committee on Child Obesity, Head Start, the WIC program, and the USDA Food and Nutrition Service. The division of responsibility in feeding model, or the DOR, was developed by Ellen Satter, who was a family therapist, nutritionist, and dietician. their model for how to encourage and guide children towards a healthy relationship with food has been proven successful time and time again.

The ultimate goal of DOR model is to encourage what the Ellen Satter Institute refers to as eating competency. This is the healthy relationship in food that was mentioned earlier. With that goal in mind, it lays out guidelines for parents and caregivers to follow when feeding children, beginning in infancy.

The DOR guideline is that parents and caregivers are responsible for what toddlers are offered to eat, when toddlers are offered food, and where toddlers will be fed, and toddlers are responsible for how much and whether they will eat any of the foods that have been offered to them. This may be surprising to some, but the basic tenet here is that parents and caregivers are tasked with being sure that a variety of nutritious and healthy foods are available to their children, and they must trust that their children will know how much food they need to eat. It does require trust that our toddlers won't starve themselves, and it also requires structuring mealtimes in such a way that allows toddlers to be active participants rather than passive bystanders that are experiencing feeding as something being done to them.

There are many ways to encourage the active participation of toddlers during mealtimes and their autonomy and responsibility in feeding themselves. One way is to ensure that there is always at least one item on their plate that parents and caregivers know that the toddler will eat. Perhaps your toddler is on an apple kick and has yet to turn down an apple slice. While offering a lunchtime plate that includes slices of rotisserie chicken and cubes of white cheddar cheese that sometimes your toddler likes and sometimes your toddler doesn't, be sure to include a few slices of apple so that there is always something there that you know your toddler will eat. This is setting both parents, caregivers, and toddlers up for success.

They don't want to be in a position in which they are displeasing parents and caregivers and getting in trouble. They also don't want to be pressured to eat something they do not like or aren't in the mood for. This is no different than an adult that does not feel very hungry for lunch one day and decides to opt for a granola bar on the go vs a full, sit down meal. The idea here is to allow our toddlers to develop their own internal, intuitive sense of what their body needs; this is a significant part of a healthy relationship with food. For instance, how many adults were forced to finish everything on their plate before leaving the dinner table as children, even if their stomachs were full or they did not like what they were eating enough to continue eating it? What was the takeaway here? Beyond the economic aspect of not wanting to waste any bit of food, the message to the mind and the body is that eating isn't something that is done for nourishment, but rather a mindless task that must be completed until an arbitrary amount has been consumed, regardless of what the body wants. This isn't a healthy relationship with food, and it is reflected in our culture with many experiencing conflicted values with food such as binge-eating, comfort eating, food and calorie restriction, etc.

There are some additional methods for setting parents, caregivers, and toddlers up for success at mealtimes. Let your toddler be involved in the experience as much as possible. Perhaps you can ask your toddler what color cup they like their water in? What color napkin? What color plate? You can ask your toddler to set the table with their napkin and utensils. You can offer choices such as, "would you like to have 3 or 4 apple slices? Would you like yellow cheese or white cheese?" Be aware that there is a catch here. If you're asking your toddler to make these choices, then any of their choices must be okay and honored. Do not offer a choice between cheeses if you aren't able to or don't want to honor it. Do not offer the red cup or the green cup if the red cup is in the dishwasher, etc.

When parents and caregivers allow their toddlers to make choices around their experiences, they give them a sense of ownership and autonomy over the experience, and this contributes to a toddler's feeling of involvement and their desire to be a part of the mealtime experience. Another way to do this is to allow your toddler to eat as they would like to eat. Offer proper utensils, be sure your toddler knows how to use them if they would like to, and model how you're using them, but allow your toddler to use their fingers to pick up their avocado cubes rather than their fork. Allow your toddler to further develop those fine motor skills by picking up each individual spaghetti noodle to eat, one at a time, if that's what they want to do. Understand that mealtime is still a part of their learning and exploration! They are learning colors, textures, tastes. So many of the negative feelings and associations that parents, caregivers, and toddlers have around food and mealtimes are attached to this experience of control. Again, parents and caregivers control the what, the when, and the where of feeding, but toddlers have ultimate control over how much they eat and even if they will eat any of it at all. This is a significant part of using loving and respectful guidance in helping to shape our toddler's healthy relationship with food.

Another area that contributes to facilitating your toddler's healthy relationship with food is in providing an environment for eating that is relaxed, peaceful, and social. This small step cannot be taken lightly, because there is a significant difference in how long a toddler will be able to sit at a table surrounded by family that is talking and interacting with one another vs how long a toddler will be able to sit by themselves with a plate of food. The former is demonstrating that mealtimes are comfortable and enjoyable. The latter is demonstrating that mealtimes are a solitary event to be gotten through to get to something more interesting. There is also need for recognizing that even at a table full of family that is laughing and enjoying one another, a toddler's ability to sit still at this table for long lengths of time is simply not present for most. Removing that expectation and instead recognizing that once your toddler has stopped eating their food and is now trying to get down, they are letting you know that it is all they could handle by sitting still. All toddler behavior is communication, and this is what a squirmy, wiggly, toddler at the dinner table is telling their parents and caregivers.

Playtime

Playtime! For most adults, it's easy to associate playtime as time spent goofing off or maybe even as a waste of time, but for toddlers, it is so much more. Maria Montessori, the founder and creator of the Montessori system of schooling, famously stated that "Play is the work of the child," and this could not be true. What may look like a waste of time to an adult, is a toddler whose brain is rapidly developing and making new connections as they explore, handle, and manipulate the world around them. Play is where toddlers will learn how to interact with their world and everything in it. The wooden puzzle pieces they are working with offer an opportunity to develop their cognitive and problem-solving skills, to better develop their fine motor skills and their hand and eye coordination, and to experience the feeling of pride that helps build their self-esteem when they are finally able to put each piece where it belongs. The building block set they are using gives toddlers the opportunity to practice their fine and gross motor skills, to develop their hand and eye coordination, use their imagination and then be able to physically manipulate it into reality, and to build their engineering skills as they learn to recognize what works when building a tower and what doesn't. Shape sorters that require toddlers to place the appropriate shape through the appropriate slot encourage problem solving, spatial awareness, and perseverance, as they learn by the repetitive try-fail-try-win model. Dolls and other figurines provide tools for toddlers to engage in the imaginative play that helps them explore and reinforce what they are learning about social dynamics and interactions. A wooden spoon and a plastic mixing bowl turned upside down are a drumstick and drum set that can be used to explore sound, rhythm, and beat. Toys don't need to be fancy or store-bought. They simply need to be accessible and safe.

According to the Montessori model, play is responsible for allowing children to grow socially, build their creativity muscles, and expand and strengthen their problem-solving skills, language skills, and physical skills. The Montessori model encourages open-ended toys that may be used and manipulated by children in a variety of ways, and that encourage children to use their imagination to solve problems, cooperate with others, and engage their creativity. An example of open-ended toys would be toys like Legos and blocks that a toddler can choose what they want to do with rather than a game set with a specific set of rules that must be followed in order to engage with the game.

Toddlers often make the leap from solitary play to parallel play around the age of two. Solitary play is what babies typically do, where they can fixate on an object of interest alone and by themselves for large periods of time, without needing anyone else to interact with or engage with them. Toddlers and children much older will still engage in solitary play, but toddlers make the shift to parallel play, which is where they will play alongside their peers, but not in a way that appears that they are necessarily interacting together. They may be playing with similar toys or completely different toys, but they are playing side by side and enjoying the company of another child nearby. Group play doesn't typically develop until around the age of three. Then children are ready to being playing cooperatively and interactively, sharing and taking turns. Before then, toddlers may appear to be uninterested in playing "together," but parallel play side by side still offers social advantages for them at that time. All these forms of play are useful and healthy, and toddlers should always be allowed to pursue the form of play they are authentically drawn to at the time without being pushed into another by parents and caregivers.

As each of these forms of play have their place, the most fundamental aspect in each is that children should be allowed to develop their own play themes. Toddlers don't need their parents and caregivers to tell or show them how to play. They simply need to be provided with a safe and accessible space to explore safe and interesting toys. In fact, this is a part of the loving and respectful guidance that allows them autonomy and choice in a safe situation.

Loving our Toddlers with a Routine

Toddlers are growing and developing so quickly, and every day is full of new discoveries! While this is incredibly exciting for parents and caregivers to witness, there are times that this may be overwhelming for our precious toddlers who are going through it. A basic concept for providing a loving and respectful guidance for our toddlers during this time of great change and excitement, is to provide a constant routine.

Routine can sadly sometimes be associated with a negative perception of staleness, sameness, or a boring life. This could not be further from the truth for toddlers! For toddlers, routine provides a sense of safety and predictability, where they can understand and prepare for the next step in their day to day lives. As we discussed above, toddlers don't have much freedom and autonomy in their daily lives but having a set routine allows our toddlers to know what to expect during their days. If every day, the routine is brush teeth, read book, then lay down for bed, then the surprise of bedtime is removed every evening because your toddler is able to anticipate each next step and feel the sense of security of knowing that there is a comforting predictability and a sense of sureness to their days.

There is also an ease of mind that comes with knowing what to expect that is all too often unavailable to toddlers. They go through their days being surprised and perplexed by the world around them, surely it must be comforting for them to know what to expect every night after they brush their teeth, right?

According to Aha! Parenting magazine, there are several benefits to implementing routines. One is that it decreases power struggles because the toddler can understand what is coming next rather than being taken by surprise by what their parent/caregiver is expecting of them. This also increases cooperation and encourages our toddlers to actively participate; for example, if there is always a bedtime story after brushing teeth, then not only will our toddler be a willing participant in the teeth brushing to get to their story quicker, but they may even go to their bookshelf and pick the book they want to read without being prompted! Following a routine also allows for toddlers to learn how to look ahead; for example, if you're going to the park "after lunch," then your toddler knows that "lunch" is the event that will come before the park. They can't look at the clock to know when noon is, but they understand that lunch will be served, they will eat, and then they will go the park. This allows for a smoother transition for all.

It has also been observed that toddlers whose lives follow a predictable daily routine are more independent and engaged in their environment. When parents and caregivers provide toddlers with a daily routine, toddlers feel secure in what their days will look like and are more comfortable in reaching out to engage in their environment. This doesn't mean there can never be breaks in the routine or surprises, it just means that when these do come, our toddlers are already in a steady, secure, and comfortable place and are better equipped to deal with the unexpected.

Routine and Rest

With great routine, comes great rest! As with the rest of their days, toddlers thrive on a predictable sleep schedule. To begin, let's look at some of the toddler sleep guidelines that have been given by the American Academy of Sleep Medicine that have been endorsed by the American Academy of Pediatrics. The American Academy of Sleep Medicine recommends that children between one and two years old should sleep between eleven and fourteen hours per day (including their naps) and that children between three and five should sleep between ten to thirteen hours per day (including their naps). The American Academy of Sleep Medicine outlines several advantages to ensuring our children get an adequate amount of daily sleep, including improved behavior, learning, memory, attention, emotional regulation, and mental and physical health! That's more than enough to inspire parents and caregivers to ensure their toddlers are getting enough sleep, isn't it?

Now the question remains, how? Most parents and caregivers have experienced one or two hiccups related to sleep and their toddler, often including falling asleep and then staying asleep. It may be helpful to first ensure that parents and caregivers are viewing the process as a facilitator of helping their toddlers to get the kind of restorative and restful sleep that is so crucial during this period of intense growth and development, and also as a guide for future healthy sleep habits. This is a part of creating a firm foundation for the rest of their lives. Just as with so many of the other areas that parents and caregivers are tasked with guiding and teaching toddlers to be successful in, restful sleep is something that toddlers often blossom with the right mindset from the people they look to for guidance. This is an area that all too often results in struggle, as parents and caregivers find themselves focused on forcing an outcome rather than helping their toddlers develop healthy habits that will set them on a path to success.

In order to meet the daily suggested sleep guidelines, set by the American Academy of Sleep Medicine, toddlers will require at least one nap during their day. Many toddlers naturally wake early sometime between six and eight in the morning. It's quite common for toddlers to take their first nap just a few hours after waking up in the morning, and this can be as long as two hours long. Many toddlers then get sleepy in the afternoon and ready for a mid-afternoon nap in the two o'clock to four o'clock range, and how late parents and caregivers allow for this nap to continue will directly affect bedtime. Common bedtimes for toddlers are typically in the window of time between six and eight pm. For a toddler whose afternoon nap comes closer to the 2 o'clock time frame, they will likely be ready for bed closer to 6 o'clock, but the toddler whose afternoon nap falls closer to the 4 o'clock range, they won't likely be ready for bed until closer to the 8 o'clock time.

All of these timeframes and ranges are estimates, and every child and every family is different. As far as the exact times that will work for you, that will have to be figured out when examining family schedules. The first step in figuring out which sleep schedules will work best for your family is in determining when the ideal time is for your toddler to wake, and when is the ideal time for your toddler to go to sleep at night. Once you have these two times, you can work to structure naps within that time frame as they work for you and your family.

Working within the framework of whatever your family's ideal sleep times will be, there are a couple of different schools of thought on toddler sleep hygiene and what is necessary for our toddlers to get good sleep, and this book will discuss two of them that meet the requirements of loving, respectful discipline, the Attachment Parenting sleep guidance and the RIE sleep guidance for toddlers.

Routine and Rest, Attachment Parenting and RIE.

All parents and caregivers will need to figure out what works best for both their toddlers and their families. Some toddlers will sleep best while being gently patted on the back or sang to, and some toddlers will sleep best just being tucked in and kissed goodnight. Our toddlers are no different than we are in this regard. Some people enjoy completely dark and quiet sleep spaces, others need a nightlight and a fan going for white noise. Some people enjoy a very cold bedroom so they can snuggle in under a heavy blanket, while others like their rooms more temperate so they can sleep with a light sheet. Some people like very fluffy, full pillows while others prefer smaller pillows. Sleep is an experience where people have very specific preferences, and our toddlers will have theirs, as well. It's up to parents and caregivers to observe and pay close attention to their toddlers to see what is working best for them and what may be adjusted.

Preparing the sleep space for a calm, relaxing transition into sleep is a valuable piece to creating healthy sleep habits that will hopefully last our little ones their entire lives through. Sleep spaces should be comfortable, and one of the things that may be helpful for parents and caregivers to keep in mind when preparing the sleep space for their toddler, is how most toddlers tend to gravitate towards cozy, smaller spaces. Allowing for fluffy blankets and pillows that can be used to create a cozy nest-like experience can really help our toddlers feel like the space is custom-fitted to them, safe and secure. This is particularly true when switching from the secure boundaries of a crib with sides to an open toddler bed; parents and caregivers can ease this transition by ensuring the toddler bed is a cozy and secure space. Some toddlers find canopies and sleep tents to be especially comforting during this transition.

Some toddlers do very well with one or two of their favorite stuffed animals that can help to serve as a part of their bedtime ritual and reinforcing routine, "Okay, now we need to find your sleep time stuffy and give them a kiss goodnight.

The room that our toddlers sleep in needs to be soothing and calm. Keeping the lights very low during the transition into bedtime will help when all lights are finally turned off (a small nightlight is perfectly fine) and this will help to send the appropriate signals to our toddler's brain that it's time for rest and the sleep time hormones will be released.

Routine plays a large part in a loving and respectful transition to bedtime. Create a ritual that works well for your toddler. It is common to have a ritual that goes something like bath time, brush teeth, bedtime story, then bed. Just as the other rituals create a feeling of security and predictability, a bedtime routine is comforting and allows for our toddlers to understand what to expect and to be an active part of the process rather than a passive bystander. There are opportunities here to allow for some autonomy and choice, as well. Parents and caregivers can ask toddlers to choose between two sets of pajamas, to decide if they would like to brush their teeth first or if they would like their parent/caregiver to brush their teeth for them first, or to pick out which book they would like to read. To set your toddler up for success in their choices, it can be helpful to limit how many choices they have, between two or three items. Otherwise, they can become overwhelmed by an entire drawer of pajamas or an entire bookshelf of reading choices and the entire process can become stressful and time-consuming.

Once the bedtime ritual has been established, it should be followed as closely as possible every evening, and even naptime should have their own ritual. Perhaps it may be modified to drop the bath and the brushing of the teeth but keep the bedtime story so there is a steady cue present there that reminds the toddler that this is a regular and predictable part of your day. Often, a toddler that may be resistant to the idea of "going to sleep" or "bedtime" may do better with the cue to "rest your body" instead. Tell them that they don't have to go to sleep if they don't want to, but they do have to rest their body, and often, sleep will easily follow. If there is resistance at any point during the bedtime ritual, it's best to honestly and respectfully acknowledge it. "You are saying you do not want to brush your teeth, but it's time for us to brush. Let's brush your teeth so you can pick out your bedtime book. Would you like to brush first, or shall I?" This holds space for our toddler to have their feelings heard and their experience validated, which is often all they need to be able to move on. The same is true for the transition from crib to a "big kid bed," toddlers thrive when their feelings are heard and validated, and when their parents and caregivers give them the support they need for these big transitions.

Attachment Parenting is a parenting style that promotes the creation of strong, healthy, and secure bonds between children and their parents and primary caregivers. Attachment Parenting believes that this can be achieved by keeping children close from infancy through the toddler years, and co-sleeping is often a part of this goal. Co-sleeping may include simply setting up a sleep space in the parent's room, or it may include bedsharing. There is a strong evolutionary and physiological rationale behind co-sleeping, as it is the way that mammals have slept since the dawn of time and continue to do so in most cultures around the world. The advent of separate, contained sleep spaces such as we see in modern society with babies and toddlers in their own rooms, separated from the rest of the family, is fairly new in historical terms. For young babies, up to six months of age, there is a protective effect against SIDS that is found from sharing a sleep space, and it's hypothesized that sharing a sleep space allows for the infant to better regulate their respiratory systems to those they share a sleep space with. It is also very helpful for breastfeeding relationships to have infants sleeping nearby, as it is less disruptive to both the infant and the breastfeeding parent for night-time feeds. As babies morph into toddlers, there is no immediate desire to separate them from this co-sleeping arrangement that occurs from the arbitrary date on the calendar that marks them officially as a toddler, many toddlers are more than happy to continue on in this arrangement throughout the toddler years. If toddlers and their parents and caregivers are still happy to continue this arrangement, there is no harm in waiting until toddlers are ready to move from the shared sleep space.

Many co-sleeping families arrange their beds so they are nearby, such as having a crib "side-car" where one of the cribs sides have been removed so it can act as an extension to the main bed. That arrangement allows for the baby/toddler to have their own space but still be very close. Some co-sleeping families have a crib or toddler bed in the same room, and some opt for a "floor bed," which is often just a toddler size mattress on the floor near the main bed. These options all keep the child in the same room with their parents, and sleep is a shared event. For babies and toddlers that are co-sleeping, sometimes they might desire more cuddling and physical comfort as they are drifting off to sleep, as this is what they are used to. Co-sleeping advocates point out that this is not typically so different from what most adults enjoy, too, as most adults that share a bed with another adult also enjoy a bit of a cuddle before drifting off as well.

Parents and caregivers following Attachment Parenting principles will likely stay with their toddler as they are drifting off to sleep, perhaps patting them on the back, singing lullabies, telling stories in a low, calm voice, or even just snuggling into them and allowing them to drift off to sleep by their side.

RIE guidelines for toddler sleep are less hands-on than Attachment Parenting sleep guidelines. RIE is a philosophy that stands for Resources for Infant Educates, but the RIE principles are extended beyond infancy to toddlers and older children as well. At its core, RIE principles are founded in respect for and trust in children that they can be successful in their lives. In regards to sleep, RIE proposes that parents and caregivers place more trust in their toddlers and that once the sleep environment has been set up and the toddler has been placed in their bed, it's up to the parent/caregiver to give appropriate space to the toddler to drift off to sleep by themselves.

RIE sleep principles are sometimes confused with "cry it out" philosophy that encourages parents to let their babies and toddlers cry themselves to sleep if they are upset about being put to bed. RIE distinguishes itself from this particularly harsh theory by stating that their goal is to allow toddlers the freedom to have their big feelings and express them by crying, and to offer verbal support and encouragement assuring our toddlers that they can go to sleep.

An integral part of the RIE sleep guidelines is consistency. If a toddler makes their way from their bed into the parent's, the parent must get up and walk them back to their bed every time in order to maintain the consistency that is needed for the toddler to understand what to expect. Just as routine provides security and predictability for toddlers during their waking hours, RIE believes that this security and predictability at night is especially significant so that babies and toddlers learn they can be confident they are capable of putting themselves to sleep without needing the external assistance from parents and caregivers. RIE believes that children thrive with boundaries, and the boundaries around bedtime allow toddlers to be able to relax and unwind into sleep without angst.

RIE differs from Attachment Parenting sleep guidelines dramatically in their stance about co-sleeping. RIE does not believe co-sleeping ever sets up future healthy sleep habits and states that children should be given their own separate sleep space and to be put down to bed by themselves and left to put themselves to sleep from infancy forward. RIE sleep guidelines state that it does the child better to be a confident leader that places the child down in their bed and then trusts them to learn how to settle themselves down. RIE believes that some crying taking place at bedtime is a necessary part of the process in decompressing from their day and also functions as their communication to their parents and caregivers that they have big feelings around the experience, but that a part of trusting them and equipping them with tools for future healthy sleep habits is allowing them to work through these big feelings on their own. RIE advocates that toddlers should not be left to scream themselves to sleep, but if given the space and time to get their big feelings and tears out, they will settle themselves and have learned that they are capable of doing so.

Above all, both Attachment Parenting and RIE both believe that a consistent and predictable routine help our toddlers to have a secure and comfortable relationship with bedtime. Both schools of thought encourage parents and caregivers to carefully observe what is happening with your toddler and to understand that behavior is always communication. If your toddler is screaming at the top of their lungs at bedtime each night, there is a need there that has not been met. Is there a physical issue such as acid reflux or teething that needs addressed? Does your toddler have a fear of the dark that a simple nightlight could help with? Are you rushing through the bedtime customs so quickly that your toddler feels the tension and carries it with them to bed and can't settle because they aren't sure what the tension was about? Sleep isn't something parents and caregivers have to "fix" or force, once the environment and the routine has been remedied, sleep will come. If it does not, or if intuition is telling you that something is still not quite right, please seek the advice of your pediatrician to ensure that there is not something physical that has been overlooked.

Chapter 19: Redirection to Tame Tantrums

Perhaps one of the best skills that you have on you as a parent is the ability to redirect during a tantrum. This is particularly true when you're dealing with a child that is quite young—they are throwing a fit usually due to their emotional side of their brains being on autopilot at that point in time. Your child can think in a rational, calm manner, and an ability to think emotionally—we all have this. When the emotional side is running rampant and taking control of the situation, we aren't making good decisions. We are acting in ways that are impulsive, and with that impulsiveness often comes all

sorts of other problems as well. Our decisions can wind up having all sorts of unintended repercussions that we were not ready to deal with.

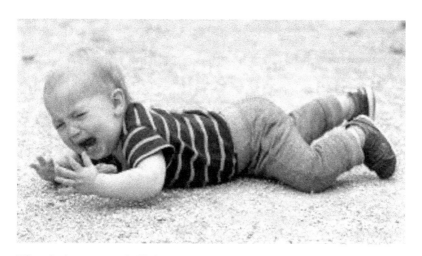

If adults can fall for these same habits, then it should come as no surprise that your child can, as well. During these periods of time when the child's emotions overwhelm them, they are unable to think with the rational parts of their minds. The emotional side has taken control during this time and is going to overwhelm their thought process and actions. This is exactly what happens in a tantrum. Your child is probably feeling some very big, very strong feelings that they do not know how to cope with, and because of that, they really struggle to make the proper progress needed to calm down.

When your child is mid-tantrum, you can usually reengage with the logical side of their mind, pulling that back to the surface rather than allowing it to be stifled by emotional impulses. This is precisely what you'll be doing when you're making use of redirection. You will be attempting to do or say something that will sort of cause the logical half of the child's mind to stop and pay attention—you want that logical half of the brain to reengage and control the individual.

There are many ways that you can redirect your child's attention. You can show them something entirely different from what they are currently focused on to sort of stop them in their tracks. You see this often with young babies-you may shake a rattle in front of them or their them in hopes of distracting from crying, or you may offer a pacifier or a bottle. Although, by the toddler years, some people stop this process of attempting to redirect. The stop attempting to redirect their children just because, at the end of the day, they expect that their older children are more capable of coping with the changes that come with growing up. Though, the tactics that you use with an infant really aren't much different than you would use with a toddler that is still learning to navigate the world around them. It will come with time, effort, and skill.

Redirection can happen in several ways as well. Primarily, however, it is the same—you will be redirecting from a negative situation into a positive one in some way, shape, or form. For example, let's say that your toddler just knocked down their blocks for the umpteenth time and is now throwing a fit. They kicked the blocks or threw one across the room. You can redirect here by trying to show something else or do something else instead. You may say, for example, "Throwing blocks hurts people. We do not throw blocks. Would you like to play cars or throw a ball outside instead?" You are not reprimanding your child. You are not shaming your child or punishing your child. You are simply calmly trying to redirect their attention instead. You are trying to convince your child, using their already limited attention span that there are several other options here that are more constructive and productive.

This ultimately works because you aren't negatively reinforcing your child—you aren't making the situation even less pleasant for your child. Rather, you're gently correcting the behavior by letting your child know that what has happened is unacceptable, and then you're offering up acceptable options instead. Not only does this help your child to learn what they can and cannot do without so much of a battle, it also allows your child to switch gears to a new activity that may be received much more positively than others would have. It allows your child to transform their anger and frustration into something more positive that is easier to deal with.

Use Positive Reinforcement

When you use positive reinforcement, you're trying to further encourage good behaviors by making sure that your child sees that they are worthwhile. Children, like most people, are typically driven by positivity. We enjoy positive interactions with ourselves and with other people, and because of that, it's important to maintain that sort of positivity as much as you can. You may have to, for example, make sure that you offer good, gentle encouragement to your child when they do something.

Positive reinforcement works by you offering a reward of some sort when your child behaves in a way that is constructive or beneficial to you and those around you. You'll do this by making sure that you're always focusing on how much you can praise anything that is positive. While many people may believe that you need harsh punishment to create a well-disciplined child, you don't actually have to. You can create that good discipline in other ways such as ensuring that, at the end of the day, your child is taught that positivity is always the best policy.

Positive reinforcement can occur in many different ways. You could, for example, offer your child heavy praise the first time they or they do something significant or that was supposed to happen. You could use positive reinforcement to give your child a reward when they do something good as well. You may, for example, offer up stickers in return for meeting expectations, rather than creating a punishment in response to not meeting them.

When you do this, you motivate your child to do what they or they need to do. Think about it—when you're told to do something, you probably don't really want to do it. You may not feel motivated to do the dishes, even though you know that you need to. Your toddler is no different. they do not want to pick up their toys because it's boring. There are other things that your child wants to do, such as playing or coloring or watching television. Anything would be better.

When this happens, the best way to approach the situation is to figure out some way that you can ensure that you encourage your child to meet expectations. You could, for example, decide that you will implement that sticker chart. You will your child and give them something they like. If they don't meet expectations, they don't get punished. They do not get told to go sit in time out. Rather, they do not get their sticker for the day, and that can be enough to motivate children to behave better in the future next time. Your child will not like having that sticker lost and will be more likely to move forward in the first place.

This works because you're primarily encouraging your child to want to do something, as opposed to teaching avoidance of something else. If you're telling your child to clean up so they won't get a time out, you'll find that all you're teaching your child to do is avoid being punished. You are teaching your child that they need to do what you are asking because they need to avoid that negativity, not because they need to do it because it needs to be done. Because of that, particularly for things that aren't the end of the world, such as not picking up blocks or other toys, you should try to step away from the punishment side. Instead, think of things as natural consequences and positive reinforcement.

Keep in mind that we aren't talking about matters of safety here—if your child does something wrong that is going to hurt someone, then you need to intervene. If you see that your child is, for example, spinning with a plastic bag over their head or playing with curtain cords, you know that you need to intervene. You know to avoid natural consequences just because they, in that instance, will be potentially irreversible. In those instances, you may need to consider negative reinforcement, but that is no longer a matter of mitigating tantrums.

When you use positive reinforcement to help mitigate tantrums, you make your child feel like cleaning and following the rules are pleasant. You make your child want to do what they are doing, and because your child wants to follow along, there should be fewer instances of tantrums. When you want to see the best possible results, you're going to want to make obedience pleasant and enjoyable.

Some examples of ways that you can add in positive reinforcement with your child include the following:

Implement a sticker chart for daily responsibilities.

Offer praise at certain increments when they are doing something—for example, offer a high five after every ten blocks that they pick up.

Offer a compliment when you catch your child doing something well.

Give a hug for completing a task.

Pay attention when your child is doing what they will do and what they should be doing.

Chapter 20: Steps and Strategies to Establish the Discipline

The discipline is synonymous with teaching and preparation, to start learning this process, it's necessary to mention the essential tools that an educator must have to carry out the process:

Weather

Interest

Desire to enjoy the challenge of educating toddlers.

With this, we realize that the most important thing is that the educator in a few words commits themself to carry out this work, since if there is no complete provision, it will be much more difficult for them to face the various difficulties that arise during the process, Since, as we have mentioned before, it is sometimes complicated. We can make many mistakes. Still, we must not give up this work that will bear significant fruits for the toddler, sometimes we will have to change some of our behaviors to achieve our goals, but this, in turn, it will help us to improve as people and not only will it be a benefit for the child but also for us as educators.

Other important points are the steps to establish the rules and limits:

Oversee the toddler.

Analyze problem situations.

Set standards.

Be consistent when applying them.

These steps are of the utmost importance since when applying discipline, it's essential to take into account as many factors as possible, and through these steps, we will be able to schematize and be objective, to find the best form of application.

To observe carefully is to look at the child with great care both when you are present and when playing alone or in the company of other people, this can indicate how the behavior is both in a group and in an individual; according to the context in which the child is, it is how it behaves, and from observation, it's possible to recognize the factors that cause good behavior or unwanted one, this will be of great help to reinforce the behaviors we want in the child or eliminate behaviors unwanted

Analyze problematic situations, and it's essential that after the detailed observation we realize how the behaviors occur, that is to find the causes, we will realize that we have correctly analyzed the situations if the solution or alternative that we applied gives favorable results. To me, it's necessary that we explain not only the conditions that give rise to problems but also the positive events, since, as I said before, it's also necessary to develop these behaviors more, on the other hand, we must also realize that the first option that comes to our mind should not always an alternative for change or maintenance. Behavior is most effective, which is why we must analyze a wide range of possibilities of the solution and the real possibility that they are exercised.

Establish norms

The establishment of standards is to let the child know how far they can get in their behavior and what is expected of him, these must be well defined, and if they are broken, they will lead to a consequence.

Consistency is of the utmost importance as it is the way to let the child know that the parents think what they say, which leads the child to teach them that their parents are aware of their behavior, being consistent gives them security, promotes order, discipline in the family, safety and will help everyone offer a better disposition, but it's also necessary before being consistent make sure that it is an ethical norm and won't harm the child.

Rules (Limits)

The rules are an approach so that the child can know what is expected of him, or how far they can get in their behavior, and this allows the child to understand how and when something should be done, the rules give the child the opportunity to Recognize between good and evil, look for things to be bright and know what can happen and when.

The rules work as a form of communication that tells the child what is expected of him, the values that their parents have and allows them to know when they has acted inconveniently or when they does the best, they can help organize and give order to the life of the child and allows to provide a role for each of the members of the group, be it the family, the school group or any group with which it relates.

To establish norms is to tell the child that we care about him, they is taught how the world around them works, and we teach them that we love them and respect him, and this way they are taught how to live with other people, the work of the norms is so that adults try to create an environment conducive for the toddler to develop.

One basis for the rules to be useful is that they are established among all the members that will impose them, in the case of the parents both must agree, these will be based on the difficulties that arise with the toddler, or to prevent unwanted behaviors.

The norms must be raised in a very conscious way and directed to specific behaviors.

Necessary characteristics for the standards

Consistency is essential rather than intensity, and the number-one thing is not to be aggressive, angry, what matters is to repeat itself so that you can learn and internalize what you are asked for; If you don't respect the rule, sometimes it is even necessary to put consequences.

The consequences must be reciprocal, and this is sanctions that are directly related to the offense, these help the child to build their own rules.

It is constant work, and it is necessary to insist and remember them every day in the same way.

They must be according to the age of the child since the characteristics of the child are an essential criterion for implementing a norm.

They should be ranked according to their importance.

They don't have to be solemn, and this can be done in a fun way through games. However, they must meet the above characteristics.

It's essential to realize that the rules must be given in advance; things should not be asked of the child who cannot comply.

The rules must be reasonable, that is, you have enough resources to carry them out, and you have enough time to achieve them.

It's essential to distinguish whether the rule is met or not.

An attitude of acceptance, affection, and respect towards the child is essential since, without this, it won't give the expected results. On the contrary, it will have adverse effects since the child needs understanding.

It is necessary to describe the rules in detail so that they are clear and precise.

How to implement rigid standards

Several aspects must be considered to ensure that the standards are practical and have the effects we expect:

The norm must be necessary for the person who sets it: This is must have an essential specific objective, and that is always respected.

The norms must be explicit: that is to say, the rules are described in detail, but in addition to this they must focus on the behavior and positively present themselves, that is, the use of "NO." The message must be specific and not general, so that it is easy to perceive. In addition, what we say must be consistent with what we do.

Also, the rule must be evident from the start and not coming out of the blue.

You must be sure that the child understood the message: It is essential to ask the child if they have understood what they are asked for, and to verify it, to repeat what they have understood.

They should be marked with affection: It's essential to use love and use a normal tone of voice and try to avoid anger since this does not usually work. It only manages to worry them, and they don't react suitably, instead rage or scream.

It is essential to present alternatives: You can give your child choices, provided they do what is asked of them. This helps you take responsibility for their actions.

Consistent: It's necessary to reinforce indefinitely if the rules are not met. In this case, perseverance is required.

The key in the whole process is perseverance and consistency, that is why we must be patient and prudent when applying any standard.

In general, discipline should be considered as a positive education, since what it seeks is the development and education of the toddler; some critical points are:

Adults are educators

Since they are a guide, which helps the child to recognize what they can do, adults are the ones that must introduce toddlers to the world and give them the necessary tools to face it. We are a model or example for them.

Toddler requires the constant presence of an adult:

They need guidance that is mainly given by parents. Teachers will also help. To ensure that they don't feel helpless and lost, instead feel love and affection, it is essential to give the child space and to integrate it as much as possible in their lives. Active parents spend time with their toddler and attend to their needs and demands, talk and spend time with them and teach them skills.

Toddler Need Unconditional Love and Acceptance.

The feeling of security and self-concept depends on the love and acceptance they receive from adults, which must be unconditional, without requirements, for the child to develop safely.

A toddler needs to be respected

Understanding children is necessary, they must be heard, cared for, not judged, or humiliated, or abused physically or emotionally. Respect them even if the misbehave a little. Respect must be mutual, reciprocated between the child and the parent.

The toddlers are different.

It is necessary to recognize that all toddlers are different and therefore have different needs from each other; also, the toddler's needs agree according to the stage of their development.

An adequate environment

It's essential to create a constant and predictable environment for toddlers, which will make them feel safer and at peace; it gives the child stability. If it's a hostile environment with constant family fights and disturbances, the child feels insecure and this has an impact on their behavior.

Teach the child to face life positively

The attitude taken towards life is essential and can be transmitted to toddler, a good example is to learn to be responsible for their actions, and make them understand that we all make mistakes, but that there are ways to remedy them and to learn from them.

Use common sense

It's useful not to remember that this is life and it requires us to act on feelings and situations. Make sure you don't get caught up in ideals and perfect scenarios depicted in stories. Just learn to accept life and calm yourself and use your mind to find solutions based on what feels right.

Discipline "More Than A Problem Solution"

The discipline in my view should not only be used to solve the problems that are presented but also used to establish characteristics that lead them to grow in a structured way, with defined objectives, including the ability to make decisions and solving problems that arise in everyday life. Therefore, it's essential to talk about a discipline where three aspects are covered:

Prevention

The objective is to establish an environment in which discipline problems are prevented and to achieve this. It is essential to involve toddlers in the three cognitive (thinking), behavioral (as acted), and affective (feelings) components.

To achieve these objectives, it is necessary to follow the following stages:

Increase self-awareness

The educator must reflect on what they are and be consistent with what they do and say.

Student awareness development

Both the authority figure and the child must interact frequently. The more you know the child, the more efficient it will be to work with them. The three-dimensional approach is interactive and takes its students into account.

Express genuine feelings

It is essential to express emotions to the child, of course, in a way that they understand according to their age. This way, they will learn to show emotions too and trust the authority figure.

Discover and recognize alternatives

You must have options on how to deal with toddlers, but it is also crucial that they adjust to the values and ideology of the adult.

The motivation for learning

It's essential to encourage the child to learn and keep them motivated.

Establishment of contracts

It is crucial to have a list of rules and consequences, and if the child is of the right age, they can take part in the planning of such laws, to feel inclusive.

Stress management is when the rules are not followed

The authority figure must know how to cope with stress and form strategies to ensure compliance with the rules, without losing their sanity.

Action

Although it's to prevent problems with discipline, sometimes it is inevitable to prevent them. So, you have to look for a way to necessarily define consequences of the actions so that they achieve their objectives. Also, it's essential to verify if these consequences provide results.

Resolution

Many times, our toddler is out of control, and it's necessary to resort to alternatives, of course, based on respect and acceptance. On many occasions the child dominates us and we must go to a specialist to assist us. Remember this when things get out of control.

It is essential to reflect on the words of Piaget and Kohlberg where they affirm that for the child to learn moral development, they must first establish the relevant rules through their own experiences, instead of being imposed upon by others. Which to me is very important since the child does not learn simply from the things we say to them but through what they feel; you can see things for yourself and that can set you free and provide you with a self-sufficient and independent life.

We can say that discipline should seek a balance between orientation and control of development, respecting the independence and self-realization of the child.

To conclude this chapter, it is essential to observe that discipline isn't a simple process and it entails many aspects that we had not previously taken into account. It has significant benefits, so it seems vital to me that we apply this to the little ones.

Chapter 21: Ignoring Tantrums Versus Raising Your Voice

There will be more than one occasion where, despite all your best intentions, you raise your voice simply to obtain your toddler's attention. In fact, if you do it very rarely, it can be extremely effective! Unfortunately, as a general approach, it will quickly lose its effectiveness and create tension in your relationship.

A toddler is suddenly free to explore the world

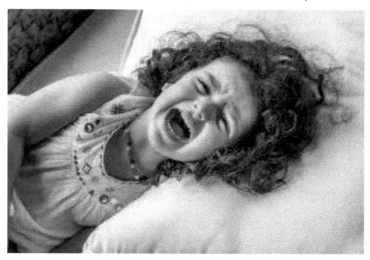

around them. They will quickly progress from a few faltering footsteps to moving quickly around the room or house. Everything they see and deal with will be exciting or frustrating; the fact that they are so young generally means that they are unable to fully control their responses which results in a breakdown. In effect, their tantrum is simply their frustration at being unable to cope with a specific situation.

Raising Your Voice

Sudden loud noises bring silence in virtually any situation, whether it's a board meeting or a toddler tantrum. The instant effect will stop the tantrum, but it is likely to be only for a moment.

A toddler will quickly register your displeasure and react to it by increasing the strength of the tantrum; this is likely even if you continue to rant and rave at them. In fact, the longer you shout at your toddler, the more likely it is that they will simply turn away. Their attention span is generally short, and your rant will have little effect on their tantrum.

Of course, shouting can result in your toddler finishing their tantrum. Although, there are several effects of this which must be considered:

Shouting Creates Shouters

If you shout at your toddler, they will assume it's acceptable to shout at others. This generally means they will shout at home, at playgroup, or at school. You will create a vicious cycle which will be very difficult to break later on in life.

Fear and Respect

It is highly likely that your toddler will fear your outbursts. While these may be effective at silencing them, they will be detrimental to your relationship in the longer term; no good parent wants their child to live in fear of them!

Self-esteem

Research suggests that shouting at a toddler will become a pattern through their childhood, and the result is often children with low self-esteem. It is thought that the shouting reduces their ability to reply to you or reason, and this can be damaging to their self-esteem although it is often not noticeable until they are older.

Shouting at your toddler is one subject that gets a huge amount of attention. Most parents and researchers agree that it offers very few if any benefits. In a perfect world, parents would never shout. However, the combination of different stress factors which you experience throughout the day can lead to an inevitable need to shout. It isn't usually done as a way to resolve an issue, rather as a knee-jerk reaction when you're at the end of your tether.

Ignoring the Tantrum

Is the alternative to shouting simply ignoring your toddler? This approach has more merit than you might at first think. The first step is recognizing that a toddler temper tantrum occurs because your toddler doesn't know how to control their emotions. Tantrums can actually be used to help enforce good behavior and help your toddler start to learn how to deal with anger.

Most parents and scientists will agree that the most effective way of dealing with a tantrum is to ignore it. There are two reasons for this:

Stops the Tantrum

Children, and particularly toddlers, will respond to how you react. The greater the reaction you offer, the more likely they will be to repeat their actions. Though, if they find that their tantrum has no discernable effect on you, they will stop and look for a different approach.

As a toddler, they are testing the boundaries, and your reaction makes a tantrum an acceptable way of getting your attention!

Little else You can Do

In most cases, there is actually very little you can do to stop the tantrum once it has started, and any form of interaction will be construed by your child as an acceptance of their tantrum. An attempt to reason with them is likely to fail as you'll need to get past the tantrum first, and even then, they may struggle to understand the reasoning techniques you are using.

Dealing with a temper tantrum is inevitable, but following these steps will help to ensure it's dealt with quickly and does not become a regular occurrence:

Tell your toddler what they are doing isn't going to get them the reward they want; you can even tell them what the consequence of their tantrum will be.

Leave them to vent. If you aren't comfortable leaving them completely, step away and keep an eye on them whilst ignoring them.

If the tantrum is in public, it's best to pick your child up and carry them to a more private place; your car or a public toilet are the best options.

If you need to say anything to them, talk in a quiet, calming voice. But ignoring them is the better approach.

You should not ignore your child if they become aggressive. In this instance, it's significant to hold them to prevent them from hurting themselves or others.

Finally, if you know what triggered the tantrum, then you can remove your toddler from the situation. You may even try distracting them with funny faces or a joke.

As soon as any temper tantrum is over, you should give your toddler a kiss and a cuddle; this will reassure them and remind them that the tantrum was unnecessary. You should never dwell on the tantrum!

Keeping the Peace

It's important to recognize that there are times when you simply need to keep the peace. A good example of this is to anticipate when a tantrum is likely to happen and diffuse the situation before it becomes a reality. This will ensure everyone remains happy!

There are several ways to reduce the risk of a tantrum:

Planning

It's a proven fact that most tantrums happen when your child is tired or hungry. Toddlers generally still require a nap during the daytime, and it's important to enforce this. You should also plan mealtimes or have snacks with you to ensure they are happy waiting while you prepare food.

Planning can ensure your toddler does not feel hungry or is tired; this means they are less likely to become frustrated and experience a tantrum.

Another good example of planning is to look at the list of things you want to achieve and make a conscious decision not to do all of them if you know your child is starting to get tired.

Connecting

Simply having a solid connection between you and your child will help to ensure they behave appropriately and can also prevent them from having a tantrum. This is especially relevant if you have been at work all day. Your toddler will be excited to see you and disappointed if you don't spend time with them; this can lead them to become frustrated and have a tantrum.

It is, hence, beneficial to spend time connecting with your child as this will prevent the frustration from gathering in the first place.

Bartering

An important way to eliminate tantrums is to reason with your toddler. They are trying to place their mark on the world around them, and tantrums usually happen because they cannot have what they want. So, when your toddler wants something, acknowledge that they have a need. You can then allow them their demand provided they prove themselves first.

You can also make it feel natural, for example, if they want a specific toy that a sibling has, then make it part of a game to get the toy. This will encourage sharing and prevent them from getting frustrated.

It is essential to keep your phrases short when doing this as it will help ensure your toddler understands you.

Examine the Anger

You may be able to do this before the tantrum starts. If this isn't the case, then you should wait until a few hours after it has finished by simply asking your toddler what is causing them to be angry. If they can focus and share those thoughts, their anger will disappear. They will also learn to confront a range of feelings; something that most people struggle with!

Keep Them Safe

If you have managed to diffuse the situation before the tantrum, there is a good chance that your toddler will become tearful. You should not question these tears. If they will allow you to hold them, then you should do so. If not, simply stay close to them as this will reassure them.

Conclusion

There is no doubt that raising a child is hard. When they are babies, they may require much of your time for feeding and cuddles. But, once they become toddlers, they will reach a whole new level. This is more than just gaining the ability to move around; a toddler is naturally curious and has no real knowledge of the dangers they will face, so it's essential for you to guide them and lead by example.

As parents, we often think that social skills are something our kids will naturally pick up the more they mature. This isn't true. Ask yourself this, have you never met a man or woman you wished had some more manners? Maybe they cut you off in a grocery store line or overtook your car on the highway. Maybe they lost their temper in front of you or had poor control over their emotions. Maybe they lacked basic table manners and created an orchestra of sounds while eating with a fork and spoon or maybe irked you with the way they flossed their teeth later with a tooth-picking stick. Gross! I know right? It is in these moments that we realize the importance of good social skills.

Believe it or not but our kids are an extension of ourselves. You may have been the most modest and well-mannered child when you were young, but if your child lacks basic etiquettes, no one is going to believe that!

Besides, if you think it is something, they will learn on their own, then why not help them become aware of their existence. You don't have to force it down their throat but a basic understanding of what they are and the role they play in your life is in your job description. You may not be paid more in terms of money for that but will surely gather praises and compliments for how remarkable a parent you are to your child. Let's not forget, sometimes that is all that we need.

Learning to be responsible slowly allows one to become more autonomous, more emotionally stable, and thus more mature. In this respect, internal discipline is truly essential.

Children must be conscious from an early age that they must obey laws. Making them aware of certain boundaries within life is critical. Of course, this does not mean that home training will imitate military rigor, none of these things.

Discipline is also accountability-based. Give your children regular tasks that are easy, age-appropriate to do. Let them collect their toys from the carpet, help clean the table, or participate in cleaning the home.

Work on getting your child into good communication. They should believe they are allowed to express their opinion. But remember, that the introduced discipline takes on a partnership framework. Of course, the child can express their feelings, but you should also expect to be able to define clearly what you expect from them.

Learning how to negotiate with your child is most beneficial. Thanks to that, they won't subconsciously feel they could do the way they want. They won't get the impression they're constantly under control and pressure, and their life is a band of constant bans.

Doing so will allow them to reinforce self-esteem and self-discipline within. As a result, they will also be able to assess their behavior and learn to make responsible decisions and take the views of other family members into consideration.

Discipline and children have always been a contentious issue. There are those who still believe children should be seen and not heard, whilst others believe in free parenting, allowing their children unfettered access to the world around them. Nonetheless, every parent is different, and you'll need to adopt the approach that suits you the most.

A parent usually wants the best for their child; this is to help them grow into well-adjusted adults.

Remain calm when dealing with your toddler. This may not always be possible, but it's a goal to which you should try to adhere.

Remember that your child will mimic your actions. They are generally happiest when they make you happy, but toddlers find it very difficult to deal with frustration. They will not always be aware of whether their actions are right or wrong, and this is for you to teach them.

Discipline does not necessarily mean punishment. There have been many studies conducted which show toddlers and children respond better to positive measures than they do to negative ones. Praise and acknowledgment will always get better responses than shouting or fear.

Every parent seeks to provide their toddler with a happy and safe environment to play in and grow. To ensure this is possible, you should use the guidelines to establish discipline provided within this book. With a little personal adaption, you'll find yourself with a happy child which will ensure that you have a happy family and they have the best possible start in life.

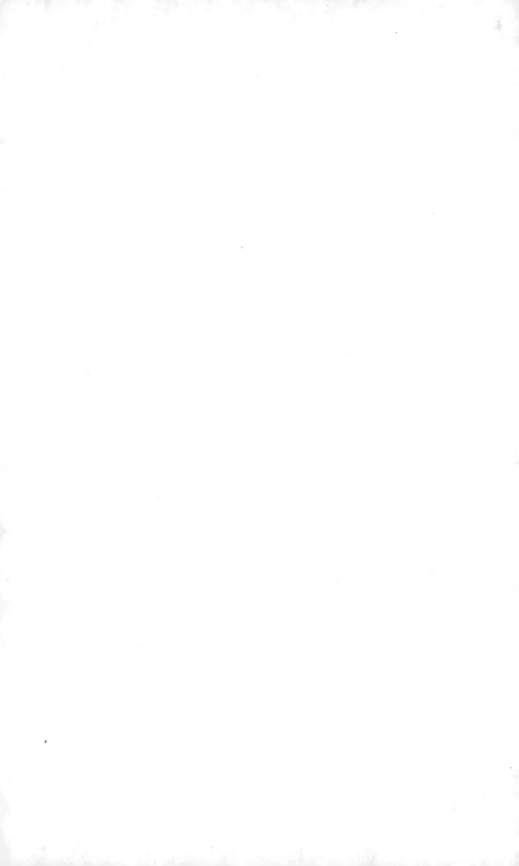

CPSIA information can be obtained
at www.ICGtesting.com
Printed in the USA
LVHW011612131020
668700LV00011B/1268